BOYS DON'
GIRLS CAN'T THROW

HOW SPORTS STARS ARE REDEFINING THE CONVERSATION AROUND MENTAL HEALTH

MARTIN NASH

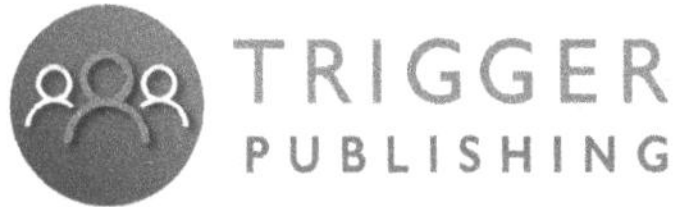

Published in 2024 by Trigger Publishing
An imprint of Shaw Callaghan Ltd

UK Office
The Stanley Building
7 Pancras Square
Kings Cross
London N1C 4AG

US Office
On Point Executive Center, Inc
3030 N Rocky Point Drive W
Suite 150
Tampa, FL 33607
www.triggerpublishing.com

A CIP catalogue record for this book is available upon request from the British Library

ISBN: 978-1-83796-078-1
eBook ISBN: 978-1-83796-079-8

Front cover design by Teresa Ferreira
Typeset by Lapiz Digital Services

BOYS DON'T CRY, GIRLS CAN'T THROW

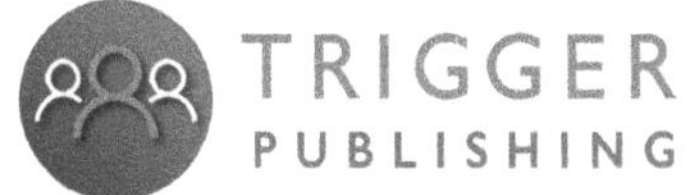

CONTENTS

INTRODUCTION

ATHLETES AND THE MENTAL HEALTH REVOLUTION

I'll let you in on a secret: I love sport, but like many of those who are compelled to write about it, I was never any good.

I only represented my school in sports that had very little interest from my fellow classmates. Rugby and cricket, I'm talking about you.

Yet, it frequently seems that it is those of us who are useless at sport that become most obsessed with it. We can't help but compare our own inadequacies to sporting greats. We marvel at their speed, agility, coordination and what appear to be God-given skills, when ours have been found to be so clearly lacking. It makes us – or at least it makes me – appreciate them even more. I have tried to dribble like Messi, dunk like Jordan, smash like Serina, and fallen woefully short each and every time.

In my youth, my lack of sporting ability was a constant source of shame and embarrassment. However, now deep into my 30s, the traditional age when sporting prowess begins to wane, I can take great comfort in the fact that I had very little to start with.

I often wonder, *What must it be like for your sporting superpower to slowly wane?* It's little wonder so many professional athletes struggle with life after retirement. They devote their lives to developing a narrow skill set, ascend to the top of their profession, then, in a blink of an eye, it's over. It would take an enormous amount of resolve to be able to simply take that in your stride.

So, in lieu of any real talent, I doubled down on my love of sport by becoming a super fan. I will gladly watch pretty much anything. Like many, I feel like my love of sport is a core pillar of my identity.

Sport is this strange sort of internal calendar. The summer of 2005 ranks as one of the greatest I've ever had. However, aside from attending a very muddy Glastonbury Festival and watching hour after hour of Ashes cricket, I can barely recall anything else I did. I can pinpoint when almost any life-event happened by orienting it to World Cups, European Championships, cricket series or Olympics...

"When did Nan have her heart attack?"

"Oh, that was definitely 2008, because the next day Usain Bolt ran a sub-9.7 in the final of the 100m at the Beijing Olympics."

I'm not sure if this is some sort of character defect, but it's absolutely how my brain works.

I personally believe that being a sports fan is a gift. I find it endlessly fascinating. Unlike most scripted drama, it consistently provides moments of unpredictability. It also acts as an amazing social lubricant. There are many people in my life, both in my friendship group and immediate family, with whom the first thing we'll talk about is almost always sport. It often fills the role of a warm-up act before we dive into anything more serious and important we need to cover.

Some of my closest friends are not sports fans – and I just don't get it. I cannot understand how they are not green with envy. Not only are they missing out on all the social advantages a passable amount of sports knowledge affords you, but also the community that surrounds it.

I am far from the first person to make this comparison, but sport and its associated rituals seem to increasingly plug communal and spiritual gaps that exist in modern society. More of us than ever live in big cities. More of us than ever before are secular. It's little wonder that we need something to fill that void. Like religion, changing the team you support is simply not an option. We are naturally drawn to the ritual that surrounds fandom, following our favourite team from the same spot on the sofa or undertaking a pre-match ritual that we think will have a genuine outcome on the match. It won't.

From a male perspective, sport also gives us an almost unique opportunity to be emotional. I'm sure we can all easily recall the image of a hyper-masculine man reduced to a blubbering mess after their favourite team got eliminated from a major sporting competition. The realm of sport gives even the toughest of men the opportunity to be uniquely emotional and vulnerable. In fact, one recent study found that male fans were more likely to cry at football than they were at the birth of a child.[1]

From a personal perspective, my own experience with sport has undergone a significant transformation over the years. I'm sure many can relate to this. Initially, sports were simply about play, but as a child, they also served as a crucial avenue for learning what society expected of me as a boy. It was where I grasped concepts like strength, skill, and learning to both win and lose. However, there were rules. Boys were supposed to be tough – showing emotions was largely discouraged. Boys didn't cry.

Engaging in sports wasn't just about physical activity for me – it was a way to connect with my friends and my father. Sports served as a common ground where we bonded and shared experiences. It was a realm primarily occupied by men, where we were taught to perceive ourselves as more naturally inclined toward competition. Girls weren't encouraged to participate. Girls didn't throw.

Even though my childhood was in the relatively recent past, it appears that today's children aren't subjected to as many restrictive and damaging stereotypes. While there are still some vocal critics, it seems like we're moving toward a world where boys can embrace their sensitive sides and girls can defy traditional, limiting preconceptions around their physical capabilities.

We're currently experiencing a significant shift in society, which I find particularly exciting. I believe the eroding of these narrow constraints are a net-positive outcome of the increased awareness and sensitivity around the importance of good mental health. Throughout this book, I will explore the collective mental health journey we have been on, specifically through the prism of sport and sportspeople. Since the dawn of the modern athlete, sportspeople have always been incredibly influential members of society. At the time of writing this book, the two most followed people on Instagram are both footballers: Cristiano Ronaldo and Lionel Messi.[2] Advertisers have known about – and exploited – the outsized influence of sportspeople for decades. Now, I believe the next step of that influence will be about driving greater acceptance and recognition of mental health issues. Former footballer and mental health advocate Clarke Carlisle has called for a "mental health revolution".[3] Thanks to the actions of a few elite sports stars, I believe that revolution is already under way.

Sport is powerful. It has a strange, irrational grip over us. It makes us lose sleep, scream, cheer, dance and cry. It has started wars and stopped them, at least for a while. We'd be foolish to underestimate its power. In fact, one might even argue that we're not utilizing its full potential.

1

THE STRANGE POWER OF SPORT

Potential Pioneers

My father and I never really spoke about our mental health until we broached the subject, indirectly at first, through a conversation about a famous sportsperson. Afterwards, we felt emboldened to weave in our own personal experiences in a much more direct way. I honestly don't think anyone or anything other than a sportsperson who we both greatly admired could have made this happen. This is why I believe in the power of sport and sportspeople to break the stigma around mental health.

As someone born in the mid-1980s, the conversation around mental health was not really on the table. This is not meant to be a criticism of my parents. A household in suburban England in the '90s who had an open dialogue around mental health issues would have been quite the outlier.

However, like many people, I have become increasingly interested in my own mental health over the past few years. There is little doubt that the conversation has exploded recently, becoming increasingly mainstream. This has also forced me into examining my own mental wellness, as well as wondering how this interacts with things I am keenly interested in, such as sports and sportspeople.

MENTAL HEALTH AND PROFESSIONAL SPORT

My ambition when I set out to write this book was to explore the current relationship between mental health and sport. I also wanted to celebrate and acknowledge how far we have come on the topic, while also highlighting that in many ways we are still at the start of our collective journey.

More than anything, I wanted to champion the incredible, almost unique power that sport has to open up the conversation around mental health. It's something that I believe is only just beginning to be recognized, and perhaps something that has incredible untapped potential. This is particularly true for men, who die by suicide at significantly higher rates than women. According to the World Health Organization, more than 700,000 people die by suicide every year, making it the tenth leading cause of death globally.[4] Suicide is driven by a complex web of factors, but it is far too often the result of societal pressure, which makes men feel unable to show weakness or vulnerability. This trend closely mirrors traditional sporting culture and environments.

Thankfully, in both sport and society, we are making some progress, but this can be frustratingly slow at times. Yet, purely from a practical perspective, it seems almost painfully obvious that good mental health will be beneficial to overall sporting performance. So, the promotion of mental wellness is something that should not only be embraced for the societal benefits, but also for the advancement of athletes and the clubs and teams they represent.

MENTALLY WEAK OR SUBOPTIMAL ENVIRONMENT?

When I was growing up, mental health in sport was spoken about almost euphemistically. People would often talk about highly talented sportspeople who didn't fulfil their potential as "mentally weak" or "lacking bottle", insinuating that something in their character was holding them back. In reality, the cut-throat, alpha nature of sport in the 20th and early 21st centuries was structurally biased to a certain kind of character. You could argue that some of the greatest athletes of previous eras may never have been discovered because sport was not structured to get the best out of them. It is my hope that sport will embrace the diverse and broad range of personality types that exist. The result will surely be net positive. Sport itself will become more inclusive and, in turn, tap into an even wider player pool, helping to drive even greater quality of on-field performance.

Thankfully, there is growing evidence that we are slowly but surely becoming more nuanced and accepting in our opinions of professional athletes and mental health as a whole. Mental health, like many wider societal trends, becomes reflected in sport. It then becomes a positive feedback loop and a vehicle to drive progress in wider society. In the same way, in the past, sport has been a vehicle for other forms of social progress. Take improved racial justice, for example. Simon Barnes of *The Times* reflected on this around the time of the first election victory of Barack Obama.

> *"He [Obama] also has a debt to the great American athletes across the 20th century. Sport not only reflects*

society, but it is also a significant force in changing it. The road that led to the election of Obama has Black athletes as its milestones, but sport was also one of the bulldozers that shaped it... Sport is perhaps the closest thing we have as a public and objective measure of worth. There was no on-the-other-hand and look-at-it-this-way when Louis smashed Schmeling or when Gibson walloped her way to victory in five grand-slam tournaments. Sometimes Blacks are better than whites; and no one can duck that truth."[5]

Another example is Jack Johnson, who became the first African American world heavyweight boxing champion (1908–15). Johnson needed to travel to Sydney, Australia, for the chance to fight for the heavyweight title, as boxing was still segregated in his home country. By any measure Jack Johnson was an extraordinary individual. His impact stretched far beyond the confines of the ring, particularly in challenging societal norms and racial prejudice.

In the ring Johnson was renowned for his grace, speed and tactical brilliance. He is often credited as bringing new dimensions to the sport. His mastery inside the ring laid the foundation for the evolution of boxing, where skill and strategy prevailed over brute force alone.

However, it was his behaviour outside the ring that drove his notoriety. His disregard for "societal norms" of the time enraged bigots across America. He flaunted his wealth and openly pursued relationships with white women. The US, remember, was a country that was still more than half a century away from the end of segregation. His mere existence as an unapologetically successful Black man presented a direct affront to the white supremacist ideals of the era. Johnson also indulged in extravagant pursuits, embracing a world of lavish parties, top-of-the-range cars and vibrant nightlife – behaviour that would be considered unremarkable for a professional athlete today.

Unfortunately, prejudices are deeply ingrained. These biases and preconceived notions are often formed and reinforced through socialization, cultural norms, personal experiences and historical factors. Overcoming prejudices and eliminating them from society is a complex and gradual process that can take generations.

I believe sport is a powerful vehicle to open conversations around mental health that otherwise may go ignored or unexplored. I am also optimistic that this path will prove to be less challenging than the arduous journey we have endured in addressing race relations.

WHY ATHLETES SHOULD BE AT THE VANGUARD OF A MENTAL HEALTH REVOLUTION

I believe professional athletes enjoy a platform that provides them with an extraordinary influence and an almost unique opportunity to open a dialogue around mental health. This is by no means intended as an alternative to the mental health provisions that are provided by the government and health services. I merely believe that athletes can play a significant role in a complex ecosystem.

As a species, we are attuned to stories that focus on individuals. That is precisely why charity campaigns tend to hone in on a single person's story, rather than bombarding their audience with mind-boggling and abstract statistics that leave potential donors cold. We are also hardwired as social animals to follow the lead of those around us, seeking cues and guidance from our peers and role models.

CIGARETTES TO SNEAKERS – ATHLETES ARE BIG BUSINESS

The influence that athletes have is enormous. This is something that has been tapped into commercially for as long as anyone can remember. Way back in 1875, the US-based tobacco company Allen and Ginter released its first set of cigarette cards. Each pack contained a card depicting celebrities of the day, and among them were baseball players and boxers. They were an instant hit, and other tobacco companies in the US and UK quickly followed suit, soon making them a worldwide phenomenon. They were essentially the forerunners of the multi-billion-pound trading card industry. However, they revealed a truth that stands to this very day: association with sportspeople is very good for business..

There are, of course, countless examples in the field of athlete-led marketing; however, few partnerships have been as transformative as the one between basketball legend Michael Jordan and sportswear giant Nike. The convergence of Jordan's unparalleled on-court prowess and Nike's innovative marketing strategies forever altered the landscape of both sports and business.

In the mid-1980s, Nike was a mid-level running shoe brand grappling with the challenge of carving out a distinct identity in an increasingly competitive sportswear market. Enter Michael Jordan, a highly ranked draft pick who was earmarked for greatness in the NBA. Recognizing the immense potential, Nike embarked on a groundbreaking partnership with Jordan, resulting in the launch of the first Air Jordan sneaker in 1985.

The Air Jordan brand was more than just a sneaker – it was a cultural phenomenon that transcended the boundaries of sports. The iconic "Be Like Mike" campaign encapsulated the aspirational nature of the brand, inspiring countless individuals to not only emulate his basketball skills, but also adopt his relentless work ethic.

As Air Jordans flew off the shelves, Nike's fortunes soared to unprecedented heights. The collaboration with Jordan turned out to be a colossal financial success, with the Air Jordan line consistently contributing a substantial portion of Nike's revenue. This partnership not only propelled Nike to the top of the sportswear industry, but also secured Michael Jordan's legacy as one of the most influential athletes in the world.

In their initial predictions, Nike hoped Jordan would generate $3 million in the span of the four years of his first Nike contract. Today, Jordan generates those $3 million every five hours. Nike pays him $410,000 per day, and he earns a staggering $150 million per year. This is because of the incredible foresight that the Jordan family had in negotiating that they would receive 5 per cent of every single Air Jordan branded item sold.[6]

The influence of athletes extends far beyond commercial appeal. A recent study by the Barna Research Group found that about two-thirds of Americans think athletes have more influence on society today than professional faith leaders.[7]

This is precisely why I believe that sportspeople can play a fundamental role in helping to advance the mental health revolution. They are unquestionably some of the most influential, loved and highly respected members of our global community. In the context of the fight for the destigmatization of mental health issues, they are currently an underutilized and undervalued resource.

2

A TALE OF TWO TRAILBLAZERS

Trescothick and Fury

There are two athletes in particular who inspired me to start examining my own mental health. They are two of the most important characters on my own mental health journey. These are their stories. Yet, the ripple of their impact on generations to come could be far more profound than any of their incredible sporting achievements.

MARCUS TRESCOTHICK – A TRUE PIONEER BEYOND THE BOUNDARY ROPE

For me, it all started with Marcus Trescothick. For those not as obsessed with cricket as I am, Trescothick was a powerful opening batsman. A huge man from the west of England, for who you don't need to squint too hard to imagine his agricultural ancestors.

In 2005, Trescothick faced down the great Australian team of Shane Warne, Ricky Ponting and Glenn McGrath, considered by many to be the greatest in the history of the game. Australia were a fearsome unit who had handed out regular beatings to England in the bi-annual Ashes series throughout my childhood. Australia's domination over England was so complete that, from the perspective of this Englishman, it was less a sporting contest and more a horror show.

Trescothick was part of the team that defied the odds to regain the Ashes urn for the first time in 18 years, coming from 1–0 down to claim the series 2–1.

However, within a year, he had played his final test match.

It was a vanishingly short career for a man of his outrageous talent. The reason he gave for his initial withdrawal, which turned into permanent retirement from international cricket, was a stress-related illness.

I'm a man born in the mid-1980s with an alpha-male father from a small suburban town, like Trescothick, in the west of England. As already mentioned, mental health issues were not really discussed in my house. My paternal grandfather died by suicide when my own father was just six years old, a fact I have always been at least vaguely aware of, but that was really the extent of mental health conversations in my house.

It was treated as a black-and-white issue: you were either mentally ill, or you were okay. There was no grey in-between. I am certain this was far from an atypical childhood for people of my generation.

Boys didn't cry.

This was particularly true of sportsmen. My father played both rugby and football to a decent standard, although he fell out of love with the latter, as he became frustrated by the increased "diving" that came into the game around the 1990s. He squarely attributed the blame for this to the foreign players who were becoming increasingly common in English football.

Around this same time, Marcus Trescothick was breaking into the Somerset First XI. Trescothick's cricketing journey began when he signed his first professional contract the day after completing his GCSEs. His early years were filled with promise, and he quickly became one of the most talked-about young batsmen in the country. However, it wasn't until a seemingly insignificant county fixture in the 1999 season that his career took a pivotal turn.

Facing Duncan Fletcher's Glamorgan side at Taunton, the then 23-year-old Trescothick played a knock that would catch the eye of Fletcher, who was on the verge of taking over as the England coach. Trescothick recounts the significance of that innings, saying, "My first-class numbers were average... but then one knock changed my career."[8] Fletcher's influence on Trescothick extended beyond that crucial selection. The former England head coach played a significant role in equipping him for the demands of international cricket.

Trescothick went on to be a mainstay in the resurgent England team of the early 2000s, culminating in the pivotal Ashes victory of 2005, which sealed his name in the pantheon of great English openers. And yet, even with his career on an upward trajectory, Trescothick was struggling with the compounding effects of his debilitating stress and anxiety, which eventually led to him stepping away from international cricket altogether.

Among those with only a loose awareness of cricket, you may be forgiven for thinking that it is a gentle sport, famous for cucumber sandwiches during lunch breaks and pristine white uniforms. Yet, the pageantry surrounding the sport can mask what is a brutal contest.

Cricket is a sport laced with genuine danger – the reality of being a batsman involves a rock-hard ball being projected toward you at frightening speed and accuracy. At the very top of the game, fast bowlers can frequently hit speeds of more than 90mph, often aiming the ball at the ribs or head to draw poor shots from batsmen. In 2014, Phillip Hughes, a 25-year-old Australian batsman who was earmarked for greatness, lost his life after being struck with a ball to the neck.

On top of that, the crushing pressure to perform is only compounded by the fact that each batsman only has one chance. Once you're out, that is it, and there are approximately 11 ways of being dismissed. During Trescothick's era, English cricket was known for ruthlessly dropping any player deemed to be out of form, creating additional pressure. This was only exacerbated by the significant disparity in earnings between those playing international cricket and those in the next tier down, county cricket, adding financial strain to the equation.

So, to be a test batsman, you require nerves of steel and the reflexes to match. And yet, here was Marcus Trescothick, a man that I only knew at a distance, but greatly admired, saying he could no longer handle the pressure. I remember at the time being unable to process this information.

I almost felt betrayed.

He was doing something I would kill to do, and getting paid handsomely to do so. He was living the dream. He was living MY dream. He should have been grateful.

Obviously, in hindsight, I now recognize how wrong I was.

Trescothick describes the anxiety that still lurks within him to this very day as "the beast that lives inside."[9] He acknowledges that the beast can resurface at any time. Trescothick is candid about the extent of his past traumas, and his openness has undoubtedly helped generate a greater understanding of mental health issues in professional sports.

His groundbreaking book on depression, *Coming Back to Me*, published in 2008, sparked an enormous response. Trescothick has now lost count of the number of individuals who have reached out to express how his words have positively impacted their lives. He understands the importance of raising awareness and providing support for those who may be struggling. In his new role as batting coach and mentor for the England Test team, Trescothick has even supported team member Dom Bess with his own mental health struggles.

Trescothick's experiences have shaped his perspective, and he emphasizes the need for better understanding and acceptance of mental health challenges, arguably something he has done more to facilitate than any other athlete in England. He draws a parallel between psychological distress and physical injuries, highlighting that while a broken foot may be visible, a "bad head" remains unseen. It just makes sense that no professional athlete can bring their A-game if their mental health isn't in a good spot.

Despite his ongoing battle with depression and anxiety, Trescothick continued to play cricket outside of the pressure-cooker environment of international sport for many years. He only retired from county cricket in 2019, at the age of 43.

It's far too easy to look upon our sporting idols as superhuman. Yet, life at the very top must be a lonely place. Ultra-high-performance athletes can face battles that even those closest to them struggle to understand.

I truly believe that the honesty and bravery that Trescothick has demonstrated throughout his own personal struggles is an undervalued tool in opening up a dialogue around mental health, particularly among younger men, who are traditionally harder to engage on topics of this nature.

During the height of his battles with depression and anxiety, I have no doubt that Marcus Trescothick was conscious of how others might perceive his ordeal. He knew that many, myself included, would not understand his decision to walk away from the pinnacle of his sport. Like most sportspeople of his generation, he would have been raised to believe that showing vulnerability equated to weakness. However, without examples and role models like Marcus Trescothick, I'm not sure when, or even if, I would have first reevaluated my own prejudices about mental health.

For his fearlessness, I will always be grateful.

TYSON FURY – KNOCKDOWNS AND COMEBACKS

The second person who inspired me to start writing this book is more contemporary, and in many ways a more complicated character than Trescothick: boxing heavyweight champion Tyson Fury.

Fury has been one of the most open contemporary champions of mental health awareness. He has publicly shared the details of his battle with bipolar and depression, shining a light on the depths of despair he experienced during his two-and-a-half-year absence from sport.

After his historic victory over Wladimir Klitschko in 2015, Fury had reached the pinnacle of boxing, claiming the world heavyweight title for the first time. Much like Trescothick after winning the Ashes in 2005, Fury discovered that the comedown from success can be brutal. It also sheds some light on the human psyche and how we respond to achieving our goals. In the cases of Fury and Trescothick, they came to realize that after successfully achieving their career objectives, the payoff wasn't as gratifying as they might have imagined. For those whose life has been lived in tunnel vision, with the relentless march toward a single purpose, this feeling of unfulfillment can profoundly shake the very foundations of one's worldview.

This was the moment Fury had worked for his whole life. The achievement of a childhood dream. Very few people get to become a world champion at anything, let alone boxing heavyweight champion. This should have been the greatest moment of Tyson Fury's life. However, Fury struggled immensely with his newly earned status. He spent the next three years out of the ring.

During this time, he publicly suffered with depression, alcoholism and drug addiction. Amid the darkest days of 2016, Fury confessed to feeling utterly defeated, admitting he had given up on life.[10] Though Fury was never a slender man, his weight became a tangible manifestation of the issues he was facing. During his time away from the sport, he ballooned to more than 180kg, around 60kg more than his fighting weight. Naturally, Fury was stripped of his title for being both physically and mentally unfit to defend them in the stipulated rematch with Klitschko.

The fame and fortune that accompanied Fury's rise to heavyweight champion proved to be a double-edged sword, exacerbating his struggles with depression, substance abuse and growing public disapproval. On his darkest days, he has admitted to contemplating driving his Ferrari into a wall, but he was pulled back from the brink by thoughts of his fatherless family. Former trainer Ben Davison, who helped get Fury back into shape, recalled witnessing him nursing a bottle of tequila in an elevator at ten o'clock in the morning. It was clear that something needed to change. And change it did.

Fury attributed his initial weight gain to excessive drinking and unhealthy eating habits. It was a revelation to him that a pint of lager contained nearly 250 calories, prompting him to re-evaluate his choices. Fury, by his own admission, was regularly drinking 18 pints a day during this period.[11]

That is the equivalent to nearly 4,500 calories just from beer each day – hardly the diet of an elite athlete. However, as someone who has also used excessive drinking as a crutch to overcome social anxiety, I can at least partially relate.

Thanks to the guidance of Davison and his team, a combination of disciplined training and a revised diet became the cornerstones of Fury's physical and mental rejuvenation. The core rehabilitation team focused on gradual progress and sustainable change. Davison was initially unsure how much of a difference he could make, given the scale of the task at hand. However, their shared determination brought them to a place where a return to the ring became a possibility.

As the pounds began to melt away, Fury's confidence and determination grew. He announced his return to the ring in the summer of 2018, defeating weak opposition in Sefer Seferi and Francesco Pianeta. What then followed was the already legendary trilogy of fights against Deontay Wilder.

Wilder was the undefeated heavyweight champion. Despite lacking technical finesse, he is widely considered to be one of the most ferocious knockout artists in the history of the heavyweight division. Before stepping into the ring with Fury for the first time, Wilder had won all 40 of his fights, with 39 coming by way of knockout. No elite fighter in history had a record that came close to that.

By facing the fearsome Wilder, Fury once again had the opportunity to become heavyweight champion and complete his transformation. However, many believed it was too soon to return to the ring with such a dangerous competitor.

The first encounter between the men ended in an epic draw, although Fury largely dominated the fight. Despite his time away from the sport, his superior boxing ability allowed him to outclass the unschooled Wilder. However, Wilder produced the most stunning moment of the contest, flooring Fury with a right hand and left hook combination that sent down the 6-foot-9 giant in the 12th round. Fury looked unconscious when he hit the canvas. Yet, somehow, he managed to get to his feet and see out the last few minutes of the fight. Most observers believe Fury should have been given the decision, despite the late flurry from Wilder.

In the second and third instalments, Fury switched to a new trainer, SugarHill Steward from the legendary Kronk Gym in Detroit. Steward follows the Kronk philosophy, an aggressive front-foot style of boxing. This seemed at odds with Fury, who was known for his defensive, technical approach. However, Fury embraced the new trainer and his revised game plan. He attacked Wilder from the first bell, eventually winning both fights via stoppage.

The victories over Wilder marked the culmination of Fury's journey. It proved that he not only possessed the physical prowess to overcome a formidable opponent, but he also possessed the inner strength to battle his personal demons. Fury credits his training regime as a powerful tool in terms of managing his own mental health issues to this day. For this reason, he rarely takes breaks between training camps in the way he did earlier in his career.

At face value, the rise and fall and rise again of Tyson Fury is an inspirational story for those who also grapple with their own mental health challenges. Yet, he is an incredibly complex character.

Fury was raised within the Traveller community in the north of England, hence his fighting nickname, "The Gypsy King". His father, John Fury, was also a professional boxer and bare-knuckle fighter. In 2020, his brother Roman became the ninth member of his family to become a professional boxer. He was born to fight, and in a family of fighters, he is the best.

Despite being 6-foot-9 and a genuine colossus of a man, Fury is light-footed in the ring, incredibly nimble for a man of his size. He possesses skills and boxing fundamentals of which a much smaller fighter would be proud. This is particularly notable in a weight division where brute force and strength can overcompensate for skill and technical ability, with boxer Deontay Wilder being a prime example.

Fury is proud of his Traveller heritage. However, the deeply held views from the community can rub against modern mainstream British values, and, to be honest, my own personal beliefs.

This was particularly true in the immediate aftermath of the first Klitschko fight, when Fury faced the extreme glare of the media spotlight for the first time. During this period, Fury likened homosexuality to paedophilia, and explained that he believes the legalization of homosexuality and abortion were two of the "three things that need to be accomplished before the devil comes home."[12] Fury generated more controversy when discussing his views on women. Around the time of his first nomination for the BBC Sports Personality of The Year award, he stated that he believed "... a woman's best place is in the kitchen and on her back."[13]

In the years since those comments generated understandable backlash, Fury has largely been able to avoid controversy of this nature. Whether Fury has genuinely changed or he has simply become more media savvy is up for debate. Nevertheless, I do believe that people should be afforded the right to grow, evolve and learn, an opinion that seems to be shared by the wider sporting community, who have now largely embraced Fury after his well-publicized comeback.

Fury is a particularly important and interesting example of mental health and masculinity. He is a swirling ball of contradictions, at once ultra macho and utterly vulnerable. He seems to both play the media like a fiddle and be naive to its corrosive power. He is a truly elegant fighter who moves like his joints are lubricated with honey, despite still carrying around some excess weight on his enormous frame. It's these contradictions that draw me to Fury and make him so compelling.

One of the things that makes heavyweight boxing so fascinating is that everything can change in the blink of an eye. In an instant, a promising career can come hurtling off the rails. Perhaps no boxer personifies that more than Fury.

Yet, in showing his openness and vulnerability, Fury embodies a crucial aspect of modern masculinity. This is especially significant considering his roots in the Traveller community, where such displays may not always be common or readily accepted. His willingness to be transparent about his struggles not only breaks down stereotypes, but also acts as a beacon for others facing similar challenges.

Suicide is a deeply concerning issue affecting various communities worldwide. However, within the Traveller community, the situation is particularly alarming.

The suicide rate among Traveller men is seven times higher than the general population of the UK.[14] Despite this harrowing statistic, the UK's National Suicide Prevention Plan fails to acknowledge the unique challenges faced by these communities. Far too frequently, local and national suicide prevention plans overlook this marginalized group who are in dire need of support.

In a groundbreaking study conducted within the Traveller community, researchers found that people from this group are significantly more prone to anxiety and depression than the general population. It found more than half of Travellers reporting more than 14 days of the previous month when their mental health was not good.[15]

Despite the high risk of poor mental health among Traveller communities, they are frequently overlooked by mental health campaigns. Such campaigns often fail to represent the diverse experiences of Travellers, thereby limiting their effectiveness. Additionally, a lot of community members cannot access these campaigns because of low literacy rates and feelings of exclusion from mainstream culture. On top of that, getting mental health support can be tough. There's a lot of stigma from within the community, too: they don't always trust the services available, and cultural differences make it extremely hard for Travellers to ask for help.

The alarmingly high suicide rates within the Traveller community demands immediate attention. It is clear that suicide within this group is an endemic problem, bordering on a mental health crisis.

In this context, it must be truly radical for members of the Traveller community to witness someone like Tyson Fury speaking openly about mental health issues – Fury, the self-proclaimed "Gypsy King", standing tall at 6-foot-9, a heavyweight champion, sharing his own struggles with mental health. There's a saying that resonates deeply here: "We can't be what we can't see." Undoubtedly, there are individuals in the Traveller community who have felt empowered to seek help and support because of Fury's actions. While it's impossible to measure the exact impact, I'm certain that Fury's courage has touched countless lives, both within and beyond the Traveller community, providing solace to those grappling with their own mental health challenges.

I fully acknowledge the need for state support in the matter of mental health provision and suicide prevention.

In the UK at least, this is woefully inadequate and requires greater resources than are currently being offered. However, I also believe in the incredible power that individual stories have to shift the narrative in a meaningful way, to help bring around destigmatization and open up the dialogue that could help so many who are suffering.

One of the reasons I believe sport is almost uniquely placed to take a lead on mental health, versus other highly visible forms of entertainment, is the inherent nature of sporting competition itself. If, hypothetically, an actor or musician had suffered issues like Tyson Fury's, it's not hard to imagine that the studio systems in those industries would close in and remove that person from the mainstream. However, because sport is the closest thing we have to a genuine meritocracy, the world cannot deny its leading exponents the spotlight. Fury demands our attention because, when fit, he is one of the best. His story cannot be brushed under the carpet. If Fury uses his platform to advocate for mental health causes, the media must follow.

It's clear – the influence that sportspeople have is immense. We want to know every last detail of their lives. They can materially impact our moods, bringing us great joy and also despair. We will even buy what they tell us to, just to bask in a small piece of their reflective glory. So, if they are highly influential, then surely there are also ways in which their influence is either being undervalued or underutilized. For a century and a half, sportspeople's influence has been exploited for commercial gains. We are only just waking up to the possibility of their potential for good, namely in the field of mental health advocacy.

I also believe in the power of athletes as mental health advocates because it is what I have personally experienced. As shallow as this may sound, it wasn't until I reflected on mental wellness through the lens of individuals like Trescothick and Fury that I was able to fully address my own personal mental health struggles. This is partly because my generation was raised without the tools to navigate complex issues surrounding mental health.

Fury and Trescothick served as my initial inspiration for embarking on the journey of writing this book, yet they merely represent a piece of a much bigger story. I am convinced that the significance and potential power of athletes' contributions to the battle for better comprehension and acceptance of mental health challenges is being overlooked and neglected.

Once I started researching this book, it was clear that our attitudes toward mental health are changing and evolving all the time. There are so many brave men and women out there who are standing tall as beacons against stigmatization. I will cover just a few of them in these pages. They are all in some way helping to crack open a conversation that is vital, not just for those at the very elite level of sport, but for us all.

3

SPORT AND MENTAL HEALTH

A Chicken-or-Egg Question

As I have embarked on this journey to show the influence that athletes can have in the arena of mental health, I have returned to one question time and time again: are athletes by their very nature more prone to mental health issues than the general population?

Part of the reason this fascinates me is because those who reach the elite level of any sport are, by definition, not "normal". They have overcome seemingly impossible odds. A mix of talent, circumstance, perseverance and luck are usually required. We have also attributed something extra to those with true star quality – we sometimes refer to this as an X factor. However, as our understanding of neuroscience improves, it may one day be possible to also quantify deeper psychological traits that are more commonly found in those that excel in specific fields, such as sport.

The path to sporting greatness is strewn with obstacles that make reaching the top nearly impossible. At the highest echelons of professional sports, the competition is fierce and unforgiving.

Athletes must possess exceptional skills, unwavering dedication and a relentless work ethic to outperform their exceptional rivals consistently. The continual need for improvement and the pressure to surpass oneself creates an atmosphere where even the smallest margins of error can determine victory or defeat. Most professional sports naturally demand an extraordinary level of physical prowess. So, many athletes must endure gruelling training regimes, push their bodies to the limits and maintain peak fitness.

Reaching the top of professional sport necessitates tremendous sacrifices. Athletes must dedicate countless hours to training, leaving little time for leisure or personal commitments. Social lives may take a backseat as sportspeople prioritize their athletic pursuits. This is particularly challenging, as the peak years of development for an athlete on the cusp of greatness often coincides with the temptations of partying and peer pressures associated with adolescence.

There is no doubt about it – reaching the pinnacle of professional sports is a rare and extraordinary achievement. Athletes who stand atop the podium demonstrate exceptional skill, dedication and resilience. A dream for millions becomes the reality for only a handful.

So, the question remains: is there something in the very make-up of athletes that gives them the edge when it comes to sporting achievement? Is there something deeply ingrained within those who reach the very top, something that allows them to see past the insurmountable odds, withstand the physical toll and rise above the constant pressure to perform, the injuries, burnout and mental exhaustion?

MIND IN MOTION – THE SYMBIOTIC RELATIONSHIP OF EXERCISE AND MENTAL HEALTH

The benefits of exercise on our mental wellbeing are undeniable, and they're backed up by a wealth of scientific evidence. However, the truth is, many of us simply do not realize just how much exercise can help.

We often associate exercise with weight loss or muscle gain, but the benefits go much deeper than that. Regular exercise has been shown to reduce the symptoms of mild depression and anxiety, boost self-esteem and improve cognitive function.

One of the most well-known benefits of exercise on mental health is its ability to reduce symptoms of depression. Exercise releases endorphins, which are chemicals in the brain that make us feel good. These endorphins act as natural antidepressants, and studies have shown that in some cases, regular exercise can be as effective as medication in treating mild to moderate depression.[16]

Getting active can help ease anxiety too. When we work out, our bodies let go of tension and stress. Exercise can even dial down our levels of cortisol, a stress hormone, helping us feel calmer.

Even if you are not experiencing depression or anxiety, exercise still has the power to boost your self-esteem. When we exercise, we feel a sense of accomplishment, which can help build our confidence. Meeting exercise goals or challenges, even small ones, can raise our self-worth. Of course, the benefit of getting in shape can also make you feel better about your appearance, something which I believe should be treated as a fringe benefit of exercise, rather than the primary objective.

I am someone who has always struggled with my weight. From a young age, I knew that I was different from my peers. I was the "chubby" kid. The world seemed to offer a constant reminder that I was not living up to societal standards of beauty and fitness. These experiences took a toll on my self-esteem. However, what eventually made my exercise regime stick was not looking better, but the immense benefits in terms of the way I felt. I've always found that I have been able to maintain patterns of exercise for significantly longer when I focus on the mood-boosting properties of the activity, rather than weight loss or muscle gain. The reason for this is fairly simple: the morale boost I get from a run or going to the gym is instantaneous, whereas losing a beer belly is something that happens only very gradually over weeks and months. We are hard-wired as a species to favour instant gratification, so focusing on the immediate benefits is so much more powerful and effective.

Exercise has also been shown to improve cognitive function. Regular exercise can help to improve memory, attention and processing speed. Exercise has even been shown to increase the size of the hippocampus, a part of the brain that is responsible for memory and learning.[17]

There is no doubt about it – exercise is an incredible tool that is available to us all. There was something that professional snooker player Ronnie O'Sullivan once said in an interview that has stuck with me ever since: "If there was a pill you could take every morning, and that almost guaranteed you would be happy that day, you'd take it. Running does that for me."[18]

Like O'Sullivan, my gateway into exercise was running. There is a well-known phenomenon called "runner's high", which is a heightened state of euphoria, a rush of endorphins and a sense of wellbeing experienced during or after intense exercise. Runners describe it as a combination of bliss and clarity that can elevate your mood, and help increase motivation and productivity.

The underlying mechanism behind the runner's high lies within the release of endorphins, the body's natural painkillers and mood enhancers. During sustained physical activity, especially high-intensity exercise, the brain releases endorphins to reduce discomfort. Endorphins interact with the brain's opioid receptors, triggering a cascade of neurochemical reactions that induce a euphoric state.

So, why aren't more of us taking advantage of these benefits? For many people, the idea of exercise can be daunting. But the truth is, exercise doesn't have to be difficult or time consuming. Even just a few minutes of exercise a day can make a big difference to our mental health. Whether it's a brisk walk, a yoga class or a game of tennis, the most important thing is finding an activity that you enjoy.

In a world where mental health issues are on the rise, it's more important than ever to take care of our mental wellbeing. Exercise is a simple and effective way to do just that. It is for this precise reason that I have become so fascinated with the link between sport and mental health.

PRACTICE MAKES HEROES

We've all heard the phrase "practice makes perfect", but is there any scientific basis to this age-old adage? According to the 10,000-hour theory, there may well be.

K. Anders Ericsson's game-changing paper in *Psychological Review*, "The Role of Deliberate Practice in the Acquisition of

Expert Performance", published in 1993, has sparked fierce debate about how we become an expert in any chosen field. Ericsson's work challenges the idea that you're just born with talent, and highlights how practising in a focused way is what really gets you to the top.

Ericsson's study centred on categorizing violin players into three distinct groups. The first group comprised individuals who attained the pinnacle of excellence, securing lead chairs in renowned orchestras. The second group consisted of second-chair players, while the third group comprised talented individuals who, though not reaching orchestral levels, were still talented enough to be violin teachers.

According to the experiment conducted by Ericsson, the only factor separating the groups was the amount of practice they had undertaken. He looked across various fields, and found a pattern that suggested greater practice had a strong correlation with reaching the top of their professions.[19]

One of the most famous concepts to emerge from Ericsson's paper is the "10,000-hour rule", popularized by Malcolm Gladwell in his book *Outliers*. This rule suggests that it takes approximately 10,000 hours of deliberate practice to achieve expert-level performance in any given pursuit. However, Ericsson himself has clarified that this figure is not a fixed requirement, but rather a rough estimate, even going as far as to call the mass popularization of the theory as being based on "provocative generalization".[20] The key takeaway is that expertise requires an extensive amount of focused and purposeful practice.

Another evangelist of the theory is Matthew Syed. In his book *Bounce: The Myth of Talent and the Power of Practice,* Syed makes a convincing and impassioned case for the 10,000-hour theory, because he believes himself to be living proof. Syed, a former professional table tennis player, was three-time Commonwealth Games champion, who also represented Great Britain at multiple Olympics. Yet, Syed is modest about the root of his success. That's because, as he points out, one street in his hometown of Reading produced more elite-level table tennis players than the rest of the UK combined. Either there was something remarkable in the water, or the conditions of Syed's upbringing were optimized to encourage table tennis success.

That's not the only evidence that Syed gives when explaining his success – there were a cocktail of factors, he says. His parents, while previously showing no interest in table tennis, purchased a full-size competition-grade table, seemingly at a whim. Another stroke of luck is that Syed grew up in suburban England, meaning that he also had a garage large enough to house the table. Next, he had an older brother, who also happened to catch the table tennis bug around the same time, also going on to play to a very high standard. As such, Syed had a ready-made training partner, who was able to push him to greater and greater heights. Another stroke of fortune for the young Syed was that, at his local high school, one of his teachers happened to be one of the finest table tennis coaches in the country. Finally, he had a table tennis club in his local area, which gave each member a key and allowed them to access the facilities 24 hours a day, 365 days a year. It is this unique setting and community that Syed himself attributes to his own rise to the top of his sport.[21]

This is perhaps what is most alluring about the 10,000-hour theory. At its core, it is all about the power of practice. Syed argues that talent isn't necessarily something that we're born with, but rather something that we can cultivate through hard work and dedication. By engaging in deliberate practice, which involves pushing ourselves to the limits of our abilities, we can gradually improve our skills and become true experts in our chosen fields.

But there's more to the 10,000-hour theory than just putting in the hours. Syed also emphasizes the importance of quality practice, rather than quantity. It's not enough to simply spend 10,000 hours on a particular activity – we need to actively focus on improving our skills and making the most of each practice session. This means setting goals, seeking feedback and constantly pushing ourselves to improve.

So, is the 10,000-hour theory really all it's cracked up to be? Critics have argued that the theory oversimplifies the complex factors that contribute to success, such as natural talent, access to resources and economic factors.[22] After all, not everyone has the luxury of devoting 10,000 hours to a particular activity, and the jury is still out as to how much innate advantages allow some to progress more quickly than others – more on that later.

However, despite these criticisms, there's no denying that the 10,000-hour theory has struck a chord with many people. The idea that hard work and dedication can lead to success is a powerful one, and it's one that's been embraced by athletes, musicians and businesspeople alike. Whether or not the 10,000-hour theory is the key to success, it's clear that there's something to be said for the power of practice and the value of persistence.

IS MENTAL HEALTH DRIVING 10,000 HOURS OF PRACTICE?

Elite athletes are often held up as paragons of physical and mental health, but recent research from the University of Toronto suggests that this perception may be misplaced.

A study found that elite athletes are more likely to experience mental health disorders than the general population, with athletes in certain sports at an even higher risk.

At first glance, this finding may seem counterintuitive. After all, athletes are often seen as the embodiment of mental toughness, with their rigorous training regimes and ability to push through pain and adversity. However, the ground-breaking study revealed that the reality is far more complex.

In the study, researchers looked at the Canadian Olympic team ahead of the 2020 Summer Olympics in Tokyo, and what they found was startling. More than 40 per cent of the team met the criteria for depression, anxiety or an eating disorder. That's compared to an estimated 10 per cent of Canadians in the general population who dealt with the same mental health conditions.[23] Even based on this relatively small sample size, that is a shocking disparity.

One of the key factors contributing to athletes' increased risk of mental health disorders is the intense pressure they are under. From the pressure to perform at the highest level, to the scrutiny of fans, coaches and the media, athletes are constantly under the microscope. This can trigger common mental health issues such as stress, anxiety, depression, eating disorders and addiction. Also, these particular athletes were studied ahead of the Olympic games, perhaps the most important and stress-inducing moment of an athletes' career.

Another key factor is the culture of sports itself. In many sports, there is a degree of stoicism and a stigma attached to mental health issues. Athletes may feel pressure to keep their struggles to themselves, fearing that speaking out will be seen as a sign of weakness, or that it will negatively impact their career prospects.

The study concluded that elite athletes are particularly susceptible to depression, anxiety and obsessive-compulsive disorder (OCD), with those in certain sports at even higher risk. For example, those competing in sports that have a high risk of injury, such as gymnastics and wrestling, correlated with a higher risk of mental health issues.[24]

So, what can be done to address this issue? The study's authors argue that there needs to be a shift in the culture of sports, with mental health issues being taken just as seriously as physical injuries. This means providing athletes with increased access to mental health resources and support, and encouraging athletes to speak out about their struggles, without fear of stigma or retribution.

It stands to reason that greater resources into mental health provisions for athletes can only be a good thing. Nonetheless, I also think it is worth exploring the possibility that those with poor mental health may be drawn to practising more than a peer with a similar baseline of natural talent, even without knowing it, because of the additional mental health benefits and endorphin boosts they receive from exercise.

If working out helps to ease mild depression or anxiety, wouldn't it make sense that people dealing with these issues would be more inclined to put in their 10,000 hours of practice faster? This could lead them to master their sport more quickly than others, meaning they stand out to coaches and elite academies, putting them on the path to sporting glory. And, as we know, according to Gladwell and Syed, this could be the tipping point between becoming a professional athlete or staying just a talented amateur.

However, we must also examine the counter arguments. While many people have embraced the idea of the 10,000-hour rule, there are also those who question its validity. David Epstein is one of the most prominent voices challenging this theory, and he dives into the subject in *The Sports Gene*. In his book, Epstein explores how genetics and training both play a role in the development of top athletes.

Epstein delves into the idea that while practice usually plays a significant role in determining an individual's athletic potential, it is far from the sole factor. He discusses how a combination of genetic predispositions, environmental factors and dedicated training usually coalesce into exceptional sporting achievements.

The book challenges the 10,000-hour rule by exploring genetic advantages that seem to be prevalent in certain sports. For instance, it reveals that among Major League Baseball (MLB) players, a surprisingly high number exhibit exceptional eyesight, some far surpassing even the benchmark of 20/20 vision.[25]

Tests conducted by the Advanced Vision Therapy Center discovered something truly incredible about MLB players: their average visual acuity is about 20/13. To put it simply, this means that the typical professional baseball player can see at 20 feet what most people can only see at 13 feet. To add some perspective, it's estimated that only about 1 per cent of the general population has better than 20/20 vision. Even more impressive, the study found that around 4 per cent of players have 20/8 eyesight, which is considered to be the limit of human vision.[26]

What does all this mean? Well, it seems to suggest that having preternaturally good eyesight is very handy when it comes to hitting a small, fast-moving object with a bat.

This also likely means that even with 10,000 hours of practice, I could still only elevate myself to the level of an above-average baseball player. I am simply not armed with the raw materials necessary to make it to the very top of the game. At least now I have an excuse based in scientific evidence for my own sporting failures.

This is further backed up by the recent example of Dan McLaughlin. Dan first read about the 10,000-hour theory in *Outliers*. At the age of 30, not enjoying the direction of his life, he quit his job as a commercial photographer and decided to take on a radical challenge. He agreed to make himself a human guinea pig to the theory by setting out on 10,000 hours of dedicated practice, with the objective of becoming a professional golfer. He even worked with K Anders Ericsson to ensure his programme was suitable to help him attain his goal of joining the PGA Tour. He undoubtedly improved his game. He went from a rank of amateur to a handicap of under 6, something that only around 5 per cent of golfers will ever achieve. However, he was not good enough to qualify for the PGA – not by a long shot.[27]

Back to Epstein, who suggests that the 10,000-hour rule is really a gross simplification. In actuality, he says it could be anywhere between 7,000 and 40,000 hours. And with most sports, there is likely a certain genetic disposition that is going to be advantageous in reaching the very peak.[28] However, that doesn't quite roll off the tongue or bury itself in the public imagination in the same way that the 10,000-hour benchmark does.

Even if, like Epstein, you're not fully sold on the 10,000-hour theory, it's clear that practice plays a vital role for most top athletes. So, it makes sense that those who reap mental health benefits from exercise are inclined to put in more practice time. This not only leads to improved performance, but also opens doors to better coaching opportunities. When you add in natural advantages like height, strength or exceptional eyesight, it can create a domino effect of success.

I appreciate we are getting into chicken-or-egg territory here, but we are only just starting to scratch the surface on these issues from a scientific point of view. The findings from the Canadian Olympic Team clearly indicate an above-average level of mental health issues amongst elite athletes versus the general population. What if the fringe mental health benefits that one enjoys from exercise are exactly what is propelling some into the territory of 10,000 hours of practice?

This also raises some serious questions. Though we are seeing many sportspeople who are bravely opening up about their struggles with mental health, if we take the current benchmark that around 42 per cent of athletes suffer with a diagnosable mental disorder, then there must be countless others who are suffering in silence.

Not only can mental health champions like Marcus Trescothick and Tyson Fury have a profound impact on society, but they can also have an impact amongst their peers and fellow sportspeople. This, in turn, creates a virtuous cycle, where the culture in sport becomes increasingly open to diverse mental health experiences. As a result, fewer athletes feel alone in their struggles, and they inspire others to open up too, which helps break down the stigma surrounding mental health more generally. This is the very foundation of the athlete-led mental health revolution.

IS ELITE SPORT A TRIGGER FOR POOR MENTAL HEALTH?

The other side of the coin is the belief that the ultra-competitive world of sport can actually be a *trigger* for poor mental health. Some believe that without the stressors of elite sport, the issues that some athletes face may well have otherwise remained dormant.

The science behind this phenomenon can be understood through the diathesis-stress model, a theory commonly used by psychologists to explain mental health conditions.[29]

In simpler terms, the diathesis-stress model suggests that some people have a natural tendency toward certain conditions, which only become a problem when they encounter stressful situations. Athletes, just like anyone else, might have these tendencies toward mental health issues, but because they deal with a lot more stress on a regular basis, it can make them more likely to experience these conditions.

Former San Francisco 49ers defensive lineman Solomon Thomas offered a candid take, acknowledging, "It's like you are being judged for everything you do".[30] The constant scrutiny, evaluation and potential repercussions for your actions can be overwhelming. Athletes live under the constant pressure of being observed, measured and penalized for their behaviour, which can naturally take a toll on their mental wellbeing.

Dr Matthew Sacco, a well-known sports psychologist, suggests that the world of professional sport is a unique culture that "... serves as a pressure cooker".[31] These environments tend to celebrate qualities like toughness, perfectionism and ultra-competitiveness. This can also send the message that seeking help or taking things easy isn't acceptable. This mindset starts early, when young brains are still developing. A study done on students found that athletes in college were less likely than non-athletes to get help for their mental health issues.[32]

As scientific studies become more sophisticated and we understand more about the link between elite sport and mental health, we are likely to get an even clearer picture of the drivers of underlying issues. However, despite the immense strength required to withstand the high-pressure environment of professional sports, it's obvious that athletes are far from immune to mental health challenges. As we learn more about the roots, causes and triggers of poor mental health in athletes, our attitudes and treatment will naturally evolve with each new discovery.

Ultimately, even if there is a link between elite athletes and the 10,000-hour theory, it is probably of greater importance that we recognize the startling degree of poor mental health that exists within the athletic community as it stands. The narrative of the unflappable athlete with ice running through their veins appears to be a myth. Once we begin to deconstruct these unhelpful stories about our sporting heroes, we can recalibrate our expectations of them.

The process of writing this book has led me to think about how I unfairly judged Marcus Trescothick. I simply could not see beyond his status as a professional athlete. As I get further away from that version of myself, it becomes clearer to me that elite athletes will not be able to be at the forefront of the mental health revolution unless we as a society continue to adjust our expectations of them accordingly.

4

FROM PAST TO PRESENT

An Exploration of Progress in Mental Health

As well as championing the role that athletes can play in the mental health revolution, I believe it is also important to take stock of how far we have come. As I discussed in the previous chapters, my initial response to the news about Marcus Trescothick was, upon reflection, something I am not proud of. The situation elicited a reaction in me that was solely focused on my envy of his status as an elite sportsperson. However, with time, I've come to realize the complexity and sensitivity of such situations. When recently faced with similar scenarios, my reaction has been markedly different – more empathetic and understanding.

This is by no means a journey that I have been on alone. My shift in perspective, particularly regarding mental health, is deeply intertwined with broader societal changes. As our community and society at large have begun to open up on issues surrounding mental wellness, my own views have evolved in tandem.

In many ways it feels like we are only just starting to scratch the surface on the mental health debate. Yet, we have undeniably made significant progress in this area during my lifetime.

There are countless examples throughout the history of sport where one can't help but wonder if certain athletes could have reached even greater, sustained heights with better mental health provisions in place. Two such characters are Mike Tyson and Frank Bruno, both world-class boxers whose careers intertwined, and two men who struggled both inside and outside of the ring.

Boxing is one of the most morally ambiguous and compelling sports. It is a fascinating contradiction of brutality and poise under unimaginable pressure and the threat of real-life danger. I am absolutely fascinated by the link between mental health and sport. Boxing is particularly intriguing in this regard, too. From an outsider's perspective, you could be forgiven for thinking that you would have to be mentally unsound to step into the ring in the first place. And yet, boxing remains one of the oldest sports that still enjoys mainstream popularity today. The first recorded fight took place in 1681, nearly 200 years before the first football match.

The raw elements of the sport, in which two people compete in combat, using only their fists, can be easily understood on an almost instinctive and animalistic level. However, to master boxing requires incredible physical conditioning, skill, bravery, strength and agility. Watching two highly skilled fighters go head-to-head in the ring is an awe-inspiring experience. It can touch heights of drama not accessible in other sports or entertainment.

Boxing by its very nature is incredibly cinematic. It is no coincidence that it translates to the silver screen better than any other sport, inspiring classic films such as *Raging Bull*, *Day of the Fight* and *Rocky*, to name but a few. The inherent drama of two fighters facing off against each other in the ring, the physical and emotional toll that the sport takes on its athletes, and the intense rivalries that can develop between opponents all lend themselves to powerful storytelling. Naturally, this is also heightened by the high stakes that come with the territory of being a boxer. As Randall "Tex" Cobb eloquently put it, "If you screw things up in tennis, it's 15-love. If you screw up in boxing, it's your ass."[33]

Although authorities have put in place safety measures to protect competitors, there is always the danger that fighters may not leave the ring the same as they entered, or even at all. This should repulse us. And yet, as fans, we find it almost impossible to look away.

Despite the dangers associated with boxing, to this day it remains a great way for young people to improve their physical and mental health. Those who ascend to the very top of the sport can expect glory, adoration and several millions of dollars for a night's work. However, even at the very grass roots, boxing also teaches young people important life skills. It instils discipline, respect and structure. Boxing is a great way for people to build self-confidence. When young people participate in boxing, they learn to believe in themselves and their abilities. As they improve their skills, they feel a sense of pride and accomplishment, which can boost their self-esteem.

There are countless examples of how boxing has positively impacted lives. Just one such example is the Downtown Boxing Gym (DBG), which opened its doors in 2007. It offers free boxing training and academic tutoring to the youth of Detroit. Over the years, DBG has supported hundreds of children, achieving an impressive 100 per cent high school graduation rate amongst its participants. Many of their alumni have gone on to excel in various fields, becoming doctors, lawyers, engineers, scientists, artists and successful entrepreneurs. The programme's success is built on the principals and discipline instilled by boxing.[34]

DBG is just one of many examples worldwide, where the almost unique power of boxing has been harnessed for the betterment of the community. Yet, the sport does have a dark side. This is exemplified by the rise and fall of two of the sport's biggest stars in the '80s and '90s, two men who were let down by a lack of structure and support from within the sport.

SHADOWS OF THE PAST – UNRAVELLING IRON MIKE'S CHILDHOOD TRAUMA AND MENTAL HEALTH STRUGGLES

If you have enough of an interest to pick up a book about mental health in sport, I am going to take a punt and say that you have probably heard of Mike Tyson.

Tyson remains one of the most iconic figures in boxing history. However, due to his crimes and misdemeanours, our relationship to him as fans is complicated, to say the least. He is both the charismatic joker who appears in *The Hangover* movie, as well as a convicted rapist and self-proclaimed baddest man on the planet.

His raw power and aggressive fighting style were compelling. His showreel of brutal knockouts on his way to becoming the youngest heavyweight champion in history bestowed upon him sporting immortality. However, long before he became a household name, Tyson's life was marked by a series of turbulent events that could have derailed his future. Born in Brownsville, New York, Tyson had to overcome a tough upbringing that included poverty, crime and an unstable home life.

Tyson's mother, Lorna Mae Smith, struggled with addiction, leaving him to largely fend for himself on the streets. He found himself in trouble with the law at an early age. By the time he was 12 years old, it has been suggested that he had been arrested nearly 40 times for various crimes, including burglary, pickpocketing and robbery.

Tyson had a rough start in life, growing up amid chaos and instability. But his journey took an unexpected turn when he landed in the Tryon School for Boys, a juvenile detention centre in upstate New York. It was there that a counsellor spotted something unique in Tyson. Instead of letting him spiral further, the counsellor saw potential in him and suggested he try boxing. He quickly displayed an extraordinary talent for the sport, finding not only an outlet for his aggression, but also a sense of purpose and direction.

This period at the Tryon School proved to be transformative for Tyson in another significant way. It was here that he first crossed paths with Cus D'Amato, the legendary boxing trainer. D'Amato recognized a raw talent and ferocity in Tyson that, with the right training, could make him a world champion. Tyson was not a large heavyweight – at just 5-foot-10, he was frequently the smaller man in the ring. However, under D'Amato's guidance, he developed an aggressive style, using his low centre of gravity, speed and ferocious strength to overpower his opponents.

D'Amato didn't just shape Tyson's boxing style – he became a crucial figure in his life. Taking him in when he was just 13, D'Amato provided not only food and shelter, but also invaluable life lessons. He instilled in Tyson the importance of discipline, hard work and emotional control. Tyson often expresses his deep appreciation for D'Amato's guidance and support, acknowledging him not only as a mentor and friend, but as the driving force behind his remarkable rise to success.[35]

THE ABSENCE OF A MENTOR

The profound impact of Cus D'Amato on Mike Tyson's life and career cannot be overstated, and perhaps this influence was most acutely felt in the absence following D'Amato's death when Tyson was just 19 years old. Without his steadying presence, Tyson's life took a downturn. He almost immediately began to struggle without his mentor's guidance, which had been so crucial for keeping him focused and stable, both personally and professionally. Tyson ended up slipping back into the destructive habits of his youth. Without D'Amato as his anchor, Tyson found it tough to navigate his life both in and out of the ring.

This first came to the world's attention in 1988, when Tyson married actress Robin Givens. The marriage was short lived and marked by allegations of abuse, made by Givens during a now-infamous interview with the couple. At the time, they had not even been married for a year, but their relationship was already on the rocks, and rumours of infidelity and discord had been circulating. The couple had agreed to appear on an episode of *20/20* with Barbara Walters to clear the air, but things quickly took a turn for the worse.

During the interview, Givens described being married to the then-heavyweight champion of the world as "pure hell, worse than anything I could possibly imagine." In the interview, Givens said Tyson had an "extremely volatile temper," adding he had severe mental issues and that he had hit her.[36]

The impact of that interview was immediate and profound. Tyson's reputation was tarnished, and many of his fans began to turn against him. The accusations of domestic violence were particularly damaging, as they went against Tyson's image as a tough but fair fighter. In the weeks and months that followed, the fallout from the interview continued.

Despite the turmoil that plagued his life outside the ring, Mike Tyson maintained an aura of invincibility within it. But everything changed on 11 February 1990, during a heavyweight championship match in Tokyo. The boxing world was shocked as Tyson, the reigning champion and clear favourite, was defeated by James "Buster" Douglas. His victory, against all odds, stunned everyone and remains one of boxing's greatest upsets. It also shattered the myth of Tyson's invincibility in the process.

The contest itself was a back-and-forth affair, with both fighters landing heavy blows. Tyson knocked Douglas down in the eighth round, but he managed to get back up and continue fighting. In the tenth round, Douglas landed a series of punches that stunned Tyson, and he followed up with a powerful uppercut that knocked Tyson to the canvas. He was unable to get up before the count of ten. The world would never be the same again for "Iron Mike".

Not only was the fight's result a shock to the boxing world, it also had a profound impact on Tyson's career. Prior to the fight, Tyson had been considered almost unbeatable. He had won 33 of his previous 37 fights by knockout, but his defeat at the hands of Douglas exposed his vulnerabilities.

Tyson's reaction to the defeat was telling. In the immediate aftermath, he appeared to be in shock. He later blamed the loss on several factors, including a dispute with his promoter, Don King, and a head cold that he had been suffering. But he also acknowledged that he had not taken the fight seriously enough – he admitted that he had underestimated Douglas – and so he had not trained properly. In the months prior, he had been partying hard and struggling with substance abuse, with a growing cocaine and marijuana habit. His training suffered as a result. As such, the shocking upset underscored the profound changes Tyson had undergone, influenced heavily by fame and, crucially, the death of Cus D'Amato.

Rewind just five years earlier to Tyson's professional debut against the relatively unknown but wonderfully named Hector Mercedes. In that fight, Tyson showcased his dominance, swiftly defeating Mercedes in less than a round. However, it was his post-fight reflections that truly encapsulated his early mindset. A young and focused Tyson preached about the value of hard work and effort, asserting that his rivals lacked the same hunger to reach the pinnacle of success as he did. As he succinctly put it, "That's what separates a champion from a mediocre fighter. I don't believe in talent."[37]

A philosophy of hard work and dedication, instilled in him by D'Amato, was the cornerstone of his ascent to the top of the boxing world. Yet, by the time of the bout with Douglas, it seemed this disciplined approach – once a defining trait of Tyson's – had been completely abandoned. The Tyson who faced Douglas appeared a far cry from the young, focused fighter, who once credited his success to relentless training and mental toughness, rather than innate talent.

After the Douglas defeat, Tyson's behaviour became increasingly erratic, and he began to spiral out of control. This culminated in 1991, when he was arrested for the rape of 18-year-old Miss Black America contestant, Desiree Washington.

Tyson was found guilty and sentenced to six years in prison, temporarily ending his boxing career at the height of his dominance.

Tyson is far from blameless in this story. Much of his behaviour at the time is impossible to justify. However, it is clear that he lacked the required support network to get through the extreme changes that were happening in his life after the death of Cus D'Amato. It seems, in hindsight, that Tyson had never quite resolved the childhood trauma he had endured without a responsible adult to guide him. In the glare of the world's media, he struggled with the pressure of fame, as well as with his almost limitless wealth and power. Without D'Amato in his life, he reverted to the chaos that landed him in juvenile detention in the first place.

One cannot help but ponder how Mike Tyson's career would have played out if he were in his prime today. With all the advancements in athlete support and a stronger focus on mental health, would Tyson have fared better in a modern sporting and social environment?

In hindsight, after the death of D'Amato, Tyson had very few people who were looking out for his best interests, the same struggle that he had in childhood. As he faced public disapproval and privately battled depression, he increasingly relied on substance abuse to cope with the pain. He has even admitted to being under the influence during fights.[38] His day-to-day lived experience couldn't have been further away from the invincible persona that was presented to the world.

In more recent years, Tyson has been trying to turn his life around. He's been vocal about his struggles with addiction and mental health, using his platform to shed light on these issues. Since 2013, he's managed to stay sober and even made a comeback to the ring in 2020, facing off against Roy Jones Jr, albeit in an exhibition match.

Though Mike Tyson's story acts as a cautionary tale, and perhaps even offers hope for recovery, it ultimately shows that trauma can have a lasting impact. Tyson's difficult upbringing had lifelong consequences on his mental health. It's something he must work on and manage to this very day. His story also underscores how vital a strong support network is, even for those who appear utterly invincible.

Life is a tangled web of experiences and influences that shape who we become. Traumatic events from childhood can send ripples into our adult lives, casting shadows over our entire existence.[39] They affect everything – from the friends we choose, to the paths we take, to the way we interact with others.

It's important for us as a society to understand the importance of not just looking after our own mental health, but also making sure we prioritize the wellbeing of the next generation. This highlights the urgent need for therapy to be easily accessible and for seeking help to be seen as normal, especially for people who have been through tough experiences. If we create an atmosphere of empathy, we can support those who are dealing with the effects of such challenges and help them move forward on their path to healing and strength.

BETWEEN VICTORY AND VULNERABILITY – FRANK BRUNO'S COURAGEOUS TUSSLE WITH MENTAL HEALTH

At the same time Tyson was terrorizing the heavyweight division, Frank Bruno was capturing the hearts of not only fight fans, but of the UK mainstream too.

Bruno brought a blend of power, athleticism and almost superhuman bravery. Standing at an imposing 6-foot-3 with a muscular physique, he utilized his size and strength to dominate opponents in the ring. His punches were delivered with thunderous force, capable of inflicting significant damage. Bruno possessed a powerful jab that often served as a precursor to his devastating right hand, known for its concussive impact, which certainly contributed to 38 of his 40 victories coming by way of knockout.

Bruno lost his first world title shot against Tim Witherspoon in 1986. However, by the time the first Tyson versus Bruno fight was scheduled for Wembley Stadium in 1988, there was genuine hope amongst British fight fans that the home fighter could get the job done. Tyson still had the air of invincibility, but Bruno had improved significantly.

However, just weeks before they were scheduled to step into the ring, Tyson had a car accident that left him with serious injuries, resulting in the postponement of the fight.

The bout was eventually rescheduled for February 1989. It was now to take place in Las Vegas, so Bruno relinquished home advantage. However, it was also less than six months since Tyson had suffered head injuries in the crash. Speculation was running rife about the extent of Tyson's injuries and his ability to recover in time. Many predicted that the delay, if anything, was going to favour Bruno, and that there was no better time to be facing Tyson. The incident added a surreal dimension to an already charged atmosphere, as fans and pundits alike grappled with the uncertainty that now shrouded the impending showdown. When the two finally met in the ring, the anticipation had reached a fever pitch.

Tyson opened with his usual ultra-aggressive fast start, knocking Bruno to the canvas early in the opening exchanges of round one. Bruno recovered, and even rocked Tyson in the same round. The commentator at the time exclaimed, "It is the first time I've ever seen anything like this. Tyson is staggered."[40] However, the gulf in class between the two became evident, with Tyson securing a fifth-round technical knockout after the referee jumped in to save the resolute and brave Bruno, who was still on his feet but soaking up far too much punishment.

Yet, it proved that victories are not the sole determinant of a fighter's popularity. It seems that, sometimes, in defeat, a competitor's true character and resilience shine brightest. Bruno displayed such guts and bravery in his unsuccessful tilt at the heavyweight championship that it catapulted him to new levels of popularity and fame.

British sports fans, who are renowned for their affinity for underdogs, embraced Bruno as a true hero. After his defeat by Tyson, he was no longer just a boxer – he had become a national treasure, a beloved figure. Bruno's infectious personality, his genuine humility and his unwavering determination to bounce back from defeat resonated deeply with the public. His cultural impact goes further still. Bruno became a symbol of national pride, making him one of the very first mainstream Black British national icons, with near-universal love and appeal amongst a largely white public.

The fight with Tyson also left Bruno with a severe injury to his retina, leaving him unable to compete for nearly three years. Despite his inactivity Bruno cashed in on his newly found fame by becoming one of the most recognizable faces in the UK. This was bang in the middle of my childhood, and I would have been genuinely surprised if anyone in the country didn't know who Frank Bruno was at that time.

However, later, Bruno publicly admitted that this period was difficult for him. The inability to compete for an elite athlete is usually incredibly challenging. When this period coincides with your greatest level of public exposure, it is not hard to see how this can lead to existential questions about your worth and purpose.

When he did finally make it back to boxing, his activity outside of the ring was ruthlessly exploited by future opponents. Ahead of his third – and ultimately unsuccessful – crack at the heavyweight world championship, Bruno fought fellow Brit Lennox Lewis at the Cardiff Arms Park in Wales. In the build-up to the fight, in a particularly spikey press conference, Lewis stated that "He makes a fool of himself, dressing up in girls' clothing on television," a reference to Bruno's various appearances in drag both on TV and as pantomime dames during his period out of the ring.[41]

When you are more likely to see an athlete on light entertainment shows than in competition, it's natural for doubts to arise about their dedication to their sport, especially in a high-risk sport like boxing. Bruno also confessed that during this period, he began grappling with his own mental health. As he put it, "Boxing is the toughest and loneliest sport in the world."[42]

In his fourth and final attempt at the heavyweight championship, Bruno faced Oliver McCall. His opponent this time went further still, repeatedly calling Bruno an "Uncle Tom". The slur comes from the 19th-century novel, *Uncle Tom's Cabin*. The titular character, Uncle Tom, was a devout and long-suffering slave who remained obedient and loyal to his white master, even in the face of mistreatment. The term "Uncle Tom" has since taken on broader connotations, and is often used as a derogatory label for a Black person who is perceived to be subservient or overly deferential to white people, particularly to the detriment of their own racial or cultural group. This was a clear attack on Bruno's mainstream appeal in the UK and his devoted, largely white fanbase, who packed out stadiums and arenas for his fights.

When Bruno fought McCall, it was clearly his last world title shot. This was an era of stacked talent in the heavyweight division, including all-time greats Lennox Lewis and Evander Holyfield, as well as Mike Tyson, whose releasee from prison was on the horizon. Bruno was 34 by this time, past his prime, suffering with irreversible injuries and having to overcome the mental obstacle of having tried and failed to win the world title on three separate occasions.

However, in a gruelling contest, Bruno finally prevailed in front of his home fans at Wembley Stadium. He dominated the early stages of the fight, and with his tank completely emptied, he grimly clung on to finally claim the crown and achieve his lifelong ambition of becoming heavyweight world champion.

However, his reign was to be short-lived. His only defence came in a rematch with Tyson. The fight, which was Tyson's first since his release from prison, was allegedly signed while he was still behind bars.

Tyson unleashed a barrage of hooks and uppercuts with uncanny accuracy, catching Bruno off-guard. The force behind those punches were relentless, as if every strike was propelled by years of pent-up fury. Bruno valiantly absorbed the punishment, his unwavering resolve a testament to his spirit, but the fight was eventually called off with less than a minute of the third round complete. This brought the curtain down on Bruno's career in 1996.

For Bruno, like many elite athletes, the transition from sporting greatness to the uncharted territory of retirement proved arduous. In a candid 2003 interview with Trevor McDonald, he bared his soul, illuminating the depths of his mental health struggles. The rawness and honesty with which he discussed his battle with depression was both admirable and shocking to a public who were not used to seeing such vulnerability from their sporting stars. He said, "People kept telling me I needed help – and I was outraged. I thought it was them, not me, and that they were conspiring... I was terribly lonely and confused."[43]

Bruno, like Marcus Trescothick and Tyson Fury, has tried to use his platform as a catalyst for important conversations, encouraging others to seek help. He has been open about the fact that he was diagnosed with bipolar disorder, which plunged him into the aforementioned stretches of devastating despair, offset by periods of euphoria. This rollercoaster existence tested him and challenged his support network, ultimately leading to the end of his marriage and his sectioning under the Mental Health Act in 2003. However, it must be noted that the difference in how his struggles were received in comparison to Trescothick's and Fury's is stark. After Bruno was sectioned, *The Sun* – the tabloid newspaper with the largest circulation at the time – ran with a front page headline that read, "Bonkers Bruno Locked Up".[44] This is a shocking example of the lack of understanding and empathy surrounding mental health issues just 20 years ago.

BEYOND OPPONENTS

It is fascinating that during their careers, Bruno and Tyson were marketed as being so different from one another – one a gentle and amenable crowd pleaser, the other the self-proclaimed baddest man on the planet. One a likeable loser, the other a ruthless champion. However, in hindsight, it is clear the two men have so much in common. They have trodden similar paths and faced comparable demons.

While their paths crossed in the ring, Tyson and Bruno's stories intertwine more profoundly due to their shared experiences and mental health challenges.

Despite both men having spent time in mental health facilities, they now seem to be at greater ease in their post-retirement lives. They bear both physical and mental scars, but thankfully, it seems they've managed to overcome the worst of it.

However, the lack of support that dogged their careers – and particularly their lives post-retirement – is a wake-up call for boxing and sport in general. There also seems to be a particular vulnerability amongst athletes that compete in individual sports. The great boxing writer, historian and commentator Steve Bunce has said that very few boxers escape the sport with their money, faculties and dignity all intact. Additionally, unlike former athletes who competed as part of a team, boxers don't have that "band of brothers" with whom they can form a natural post-retirement support network. As Bruno put it, "Boxing is the loneliest sport in the world."

At long last, boxing is starting to acknowledge some of these issues via the Professional Boxers' Affiliation (PBA), which was created to assist boxers after their retirement. But to put it into perspective, the PBA wasn't established until 2022, more than *340 years* after the first fight took place.

Though it's still in its early stages and hasn't fully achieved its goals yet, the PBA recognizes the lack of support available to both retired and current boxers. Their mission is to assist boxers both during and after their careers. Recognizing the significance of financial stability, the PBA has partnered with financial planners to provide tailored advice to boxers. They're working on establishing a pension scheme funded by revenue from broadcast deals, but in the meantime, they help boxers with the transition into retirement, which, as we know, can be difficult for elite athletes to make.

The PBA also places a strong emphasis on mental health, providing round-the-clock access to hotlines and arranging counselling sessions for those in need. Additionally, they aim to educate boxers on how to identify and prevent mental health emergencies.

While the PBA's goals are admirable, they primarily focus on boxers from the UK. But there's a significant number of fighters in need of support worldwide.

If we narrow our focus to active fighters, the most recent figures count approximately 20,000 professional boxers.[45] Based on a 2019 *Forbes* report, it's estimated that only 19 fighters earn annual salaries surpassing $2 million.[46] That means just 0.09 per cent of fighters are in the highest earning bracket. Consequently, the vast majority of the remaining 99.91 per cent are barely making ends meet, or are forced to work additional jobs to sustain their careers as professional athletes. And these figures don't even include the large number of former professionals who have already retired.

This leaves us with a situation where hundreds of thousands of active and retired athletes are navigating life without a financial safety net, a circumstance known to worsen mental health issues. Take the UK, for instance, where the National Health Service lacks adequate resources for mental health support. A troubling report from mental health charity Mind revealed that more than 40 per cent of mental health trusts had staffing levels far below recommended standards. Only 14 per cent of individuals reported feeling fully supported during a crisis, and less than a third felt that staff treated them with respect and dignity.[47] Meanwhile, in the United States, another hotbed for professional boxing, there are famously no national health provisions in place at all.

It is estimated that Mike Tyson earned around $500 million during his professional boxing career, but he ended up broke and filing for bankruptcy. If even some of the most high-profile stars can leave the sport with next to nothing, what chance do those stand who never have a big payday?

Tyson and Bruno have both seemingly bounced back from their well-publicized issues and are enjoying support for their ongoing mental health battles. However, they do have a natural advantage: they are amongst the most well-known athletes to have competed in the sport, and there will likely always be someone to help them due to their celebrity status. For the 99.91 per cent who don't enjoy the same exposure or fame, there needs to be much greater support, in terms of both financial guidance and mental health provisions.

We live in a world where we have fighters, talent management, the government and multiple sport governing bodies, and nobody is doing enough. It seems that everyone else is expecting the other parties to pick up the slack, leaving a huge hole in support for the vast majority of athletes.

So, the big question lingers, would Tyson and Bruno have received better support in today's sporting and social landscape compared to 40 years ago? One might hope that Bruno's bipolar disorder could have been identified earlier. Additionally, considering the inspiring turnaround in Tyson Fury's life, it's tempting to imagine that Mike Tyson could have avoided going off the rails quite so spectacularly. However, the reality is that we still have a lot of ground to cover in terms of mental health care, financial planning and overall support for athletes, both during and after their careers.

THE INSIDIOUS NATURE OF CHILDHOOD TRAUMA

The case of Mike Tyson is especially intriguing because he has always been open about the challenges he faced in his childhood. It's possible that in the '80s and '90s, we weren't fully prepared as a culture to acknowledge how childhood trauma can affect someone later in life.

Childhood is a critical time for growth, development and the shaping of one's identity. However, we now understand that when individuals face traumatic experiences during these crucial years, the effects can last a lifetime. Childhood trauma, whether it's abuse, neglect, witnessing violence or experiencing significant loss, has the power to deeply influence our emotional, cognitive and social wellbeing well into adulthood.

In 2023, English professional footballer Dele Alli opened up about the shocking extent of his own personal childhood traumas in a raw interview with Gary Neville on Neville's podcast, *The Overlap*.

At one point Dele Alli was hailed as one of the most promising talents in English football. He burst onto the scene at a tender age, making his debut for his hometown club MK Dons when he was only 16. From there, his career was on a constant upward trajectory. He soon earned a move to the Premier League with Tottenham Hotspur. Then, his brilliance shone during England's journey to the semi-finals of the 2018 World Cup, and he played a pivotal role in Tottenham's march to the 2019 Champions League Final. At that point, Dele was just 23 years old with the world at his feet. Yet, within a couple of years, his career was on the rocks, having been loaned out to Turkish side Beşiktaş, where he made just 13 senior appearances.

The sudden loss of form was both spectacular and shocking. Many theorized that it stemmed from his treatment under previous coach Jose Mourinho. The manager seemed to single out Dele in harsh critiques captured in *All or Nothing*, an Amazon documentary that went behind the scenes of the Spurs' 2019–2020 season.

However, during his raw and honest interview with Neville in 2023, Dele revealed the true burden that had been weighing him down for all those years. He said that he had recently gone to rehab to combat an addiction to sleeping pills. In his own words, he was using prescription drugs to deal with his trauma, "rather than dealing with the root of the problems". Dele felt compelled or perhaps pressured to speak out about his issues just weeks after leaving rehab. He had been alerted that the tabloids were aware of his time in recovery, and wanting to control the narrative, he decided to address it publicly, perhaps sooner than he would have liked.

What followed were shocking revelations about the extent of the difficulties Dele suffered growing up. At the age of six, he was molested by a friend of his mother's. He then admitted that he started smoking at seven and selling drugs at eight. He was told by dealers on his estate to hide the drugs underneath a football that he always carried, as they believed that the police would not stop a small child.

Fortunately, Dele was adopted when he was 12 years old, and his new family played a crucial role in transforming his life. However, he struggled to confide in them, even though they provided him with the first real sense of security he had ever experienced. He lived in constant fear that they might also leave him one day, which motivated him to be the best version of himself. But this constant pressure led him to bury his trauma, until he eventually realized, with the help of professionals, that he could no longer ignore the toll it was taking on him.[48]

Reflecting on Dele Alli's journey, his mere loss of form is not the remarkable matter. It is the fact that he managed to ascend to the top of his sport after suffering so much in his childhood, turning his life around in a remarkably short period of time.

The interview with Neville is really tough to watch. Dele's former coach and mentor Mauricio Pochettino revealed that he couldn't bring himself to finish it, saying it was "just too painful".[49]

Gary Neville should be highly commended for how he handled the interview. He showed remarkable compassion in what was undoubtedly a difficult situation. After watching the video and checking out some social media reactions, it was really encouraging to see almost unanimous support and sympathy for Dele. In the bearpit of social media, that itself was both miraculous and heartening.

Dele also deserves a lot of credit for taking ownership of his story and acknowledging how his childhood trauma has affected him. This is the first step toward healing and preventing those effects from continuing. As fans, we should also remember that we hardly ever get the full picture of an athlete's life. So, wild criticism around something frankly as trivial as a loss of form is something we should probably avoid.

When we look at players like Dele Alli, it's easy to get caught up in their glamorous lifestyle, wealth and the admiration they receive. However, it's important not to forget the human being behind the fame. Dele's courage in sharing his struggles reminds us that there's often more depth to individuals than what we see on the surface. His honesty should encourage others to reconsider their judgements and think twice before sending hate or criticism toward public figures. By empathizing with the person behind the public persona, we can contribute to building a kinder and more understanding society that prioritizes mental wellbeing and treats every individual with respect and compassion.

Furthermore, the near-universal levels of support that Dele received in the aftermath of the interview suggests that, as a society, we're becoming more compassionate and accepting of mental health struggles. It seems self-evident that the easier we collectively make the experience of opening up about mental health for athletes, the more likely they will be to show these vulnerabilities in the first place.

Dele's openness about his struggles could be one of the most significant contributions from an athlete to the mental health movement. It also underscores the importance of our role as the general public in setting the stage for the mental health revolution to be able to flourish.

HOW MUCH PROGRESS HAVE WE REALLY MADE?

The lingering question is whether our society has genuinely shifted its stance on mental health and wellbeing. Dele Alli's case, and the widespread public support he received, hints at progress in this area. However, delving deeper into this matter, I've had discussions with various experts, including Sarah Nightingale. Sarah brings a nuanced perspective, drawing from her role as the Player Care Manager at Cardiff City Football Club.

Sarah's first-hand experience of working closely with academy players, ranging from ages 9 to 21, offers valuable insights into the current situation. While she rightly praises the significant progress that has been made in addressing mental health concerns, she remains cautious. Reflecting on her daily interactions with young academy players, she admits that "mental health is something they're accustomed to discussing and receiving education and support about." However, she also notes that there's still a long way to go before they feel truly comfortable discussing their experiences, especially in male-dominated environments. While they're not afraid of the topic itself anymore, she observes that they may still hesitate to talk about their own experiences.[50]

This brings us back to the significant impact influential figures have in breaking down these deep-set social barriers. For me, it was Marcus Trescothick, but there's also the profound influence of peers, especially at junior and academy levels. Sarah shared that boys under her care often come in clusters, typically recommended by one of their teammates. She explained, "Some of them will ask to see you, or ask for a one-on-one session after a workshop, but it's often because someone has visited me, spoken to his friends and said, 'It was *really good*.' Then another will come, and that's how it tends to build. Once you've got one person on board, the rest will follow."[51] This effect is particularly strong when that person is a high-status member of the group. In exactly the same way, elite athletes, as high-status members of society, are opening up the mental health debate more generally.

OLYMPIC LEGACY

One cautionary tale that keeps me grounded regarding the pace of societal progress on accepting mental health issues is the treatment of American gymnast Simone Biles.

Biles' decision to withdraw from multiple events at the 2020 Tokyo Olympics, including the all-around competition and individual apparatus finals, sent shockwaves through the sporting world. As the most decorated gymnast in history, her absence was keenly felt. However, what was even more remarkable than her withdrawal from the competition was the reason behind it. Biles openly stated that she needed to prioritize her mental wellbeing, citing struggles with the "twisties", a dangerous phenomenon where gymnasts lose their spatial awareness mid-air.

Despite receiving support from many sources, there was notable backlash too. Henry Cejudo, a former Olympic gold medallist, said Biles needed "a nice kick in the arse."[52] British TV host and columnist Piers Morgan called her "selfish" and said she had let down her teammates.[53]

In an era marked by deepening divisions and polarized viewpoints, finding agreement on important matters has become harder than ever. Some media personalities, like Morgan, thrive on stirring up controversy even on topics they're not truly invested in, just to stay relevant in the media. Do we honestly believe he genuinely cares whether Simone Biles competes in the Olympics? Yet, we're stuck in a world where politics and social issues are filled with disagreement and tension, making it increasingly tough to find common understanding. This is perhaps the biggest singular challenge of the mental health revolution.

HOPE OVER HATE

If we compare the public and media reaction to the struggles of Frank Bruno verses Dele Alli, it seems we've made strides in terms of our acceptance and empathy around mental health issues.

Yet, we still reside in a society where young men, especially in male-dominated environments like sports teams, remain hesitant to display vulnerability. I know I felt a similar degree of pressure to conform to prescribed masculinity when I was growing up, and I was nowhere near an elite sporting academy. Also, as long as only a few brave outliers are willing to openly discuss their mental health struggles, it will naturally remain outside the norm. Until we break this stigma and normalize conversations about mental health, we'll likely see ongoing reluctance for people to open up and display vulnerability. Regrettably, this will only perpetuate the cycle and reinforce these problems for future generations. While we've made significant strides, the journey ahead remains frustratingly slow and challenging. But it seems that with more and more high-profile individuals courageously sharing their everyday mental health battles, progress is starting to accelerate and gain momentum.

5

UNDER PRESSURE

An Inevitable Part of Elite Sport?

As sports fans, we inherently grasp the intense pressure that athletes endure throughout their careers. Every performance is laden with pressure. They navigate the weight of relentless media scrutiny and the towering expectations of supporters. They confront health risks stemming from injuries and the strain of financial obligations. Negotiating contracts and securing brand endorsements can also add another layer of stress. These demands often result in time constraints, forcing athletes to juggle training, competitions, travel, media obligations and their personal lives. Pressure becomes an inseparable part of their daily existence. In this chapter, I will delve into the various pressures athletes face, and how these challenges are changing over time.

The life of a superstar athlete no doubt appears glamorous from an outsider's point of view, but it doesn't take a wild leap of imagination to understand quite how suffocating and stressful this lifestyle could be. The intense scrutiny has driven some sportspeople to speak out on the pressure of their increasingly unforgiving schedules. Just like anyone else, athletes can experience burnout too. Perhaps surprisingly, research from the American College of Sports

Medicine revealed that 35 per cent of professional athletes have dealt with burnout.[54] Interestingly, this statistic is quite close to findings from a study on the general population, indicating that about 42 per cent of us regular folks have also faced burnout at some point.[55]

I happen to believe that a world in which more than a third of the population are suffering from burnout is a situation that cannot be sustainable. This chapter delves into how some athletes are pushing back against the pressures of the modern world. In doing so, they are setting an example that the rest of us should learn to follow. It seems when it comes to the stresses of modern life, we are not so different from our heroes.

LEAVE IT ALL ON THE COURT

Performance pressure can be a significant factor contributing to the struggle athletes face in maintaining good mental health. From a young age, sportspeople are subjected to immense pressure to excel, which often persists throughout their careers.

Reflecting on my own experiences at the age when many athletes begin to rise to prominence, it became apparent that I, like many others, would have been ill-prepared to cope with the relentless and often merciless demands placed upon individuals in the world of sports. The pressure they endure is something that tests their resilience and mental fortitude in ways that are difficult for most outsiders to fully comprehend.

This pressure has been linked to high dropout rates – up to 35 per cent per year – among developing athletes.[56] As mentioned before, engaging in sports can play a crucial role in promoting and maintaining positive mental wellbeing. Hence, I am naturally highly critical of any environment that drives anyone to give up sport entirely.

IT DOESN'T GET EASIER FOR THOSE WHO MAKE IT

Professional athletes by their very nature are high-achieving individuals who strive for perfection in their chosen field. However, even for the fiercest of competitors, the stress and external pressures can weigh heavily on their mental, physical and emotional wellbeing. The sporting environment, which is inherently outcome-based, places significant emphasis on wins and losses. While it may be challenging to eliminate the outcome-based culture entirely, there is an opportunity to shift how pressure is managed and perceived, particularly amongst younger competitors in developmental and age-group sports.

Pressure to perform is a double-edged sword. While some can harness it and thrive, for others it can lead to overthinking and decreased performance in critical moments. New findings are beginning to emerge, revealing that the constant stress elite athletes face might be linked to mental health challenges. Research has shown that enduring stress can disrupt the release of glutamate, a neurotransmitter in the brain. Such disruptions could play a role in certain mental health issues and cause lasting changes to neurological function.[57]

So, what can we do to mitigate the risks of damaging the mental health of athletes? What steps can we take to support athletes' mental wellbeing? And how are the pressures of being an elite athlete evolving over time? The better we comprehend these issues, the more effectively we can harness the incredible potential that athletes possess to spearhead the mental health revolution.

ALONE IN THE ARENA – NAVIGATING THE PRESSURE OF SOLO SPORTS

I would describe Ronnie O'Sullivan as the Michael Jordan of snooker, but that might be doing a disservice to Ronnie O'Sullivan. While the term "genius" is frequently thrown around in the realm of professional sports, few sportspeople truly embody it to the extent of O'Sullivan. In fact, it's difficult to think of another sportsperson who has been consistently labelled with the g-word by both peers and commentators as frequently.

Ronnie O'Sullivan's illustrious career is punctuated by an impressive array of records that underscore his unparalleled dominance in snooker. With a staggering 41 ranking event titles to his name, he stands as the most successful player in the history of the sport. In 2019, he became the first player to have reached 1,000 career centuries, and he has more maximum breaks than any other player.

However, the records only tell part of the story. Beyond the impressive tally of titles lies a quality that sets Ronnie O'Sullivan apart from the rest, an intangible essence possessed only by few. O'Sullivan's mastery of snooker transcends statistics. He blends finesse, speed, power and precision. When on form, O'Sullivan is in a league of his own – he is not just a champion, but a virtuoso of the sport.

Renowned for his flamboyant style, O'Sullivan captivates audiences with his remarkable speed and shot-making prowess. Nowhere was this more evident than during his legendary performance at the 1997 World Championship. At just 21 years old, he had already etched his name in the annals of snooker history by scoring the fastest-recorded 147-break, against Mick Price. A 147-break is the highest possible score in a single frame of snooker, achieved only by potting all 15 red balls with 15 black balls, followed by all six coloured balls in sequence. It requires extraordinary skill, precision and concentration, as each shot must be perfectly executed. The difficulty lies in the need for flawless positioning, accurate potting, and strategic planning throughout the entire sequence. O'Sullivan's masterful execution of the maximum break in a mere five minutes and eight seconds remains an almost mythical benchmark in the sport.

To put O'Sullivan's feat into perspective, it's important to note that at the time of writing, fewer than 200 maximum breaks have been achieved in the entire history of snooker. It is considered one of the most difficult accomplishments in all of sport. The majority of professional players will never make a 147-break in competition. Also, a maximum break typically takes between 10 to 14 minutes to complete. O'Sullivan achieved this in just over 5 minutes. His record-setting performance in 1997 is an example of his sheer brilliance, and stands as one of those rare sporting feats that feels like it may never be bettered.

Despite being adored by fans and peers alike, and boasting a trophy cabinet filled to the brim, Ronnie O'Sullivan's life has been far from simple. In 1992, his world was turned upside down when his father was convicted of murder and given a life sentence. This deeply traumatic event cast a dark cloud over O'Sullivan's early years, greatly affecting his family and influencing his personal journey.

Adding to the tumultuousness of his life, in 1996, O'Sullivan faced another crisis when his mother was sentenced to a year in prison for tax evasion. This left O'Sullivan, at the young age of 20, shouldering the responsibility of caring for his 8-year-old sister amid the upheaval caused by the imprisonment of both his parents. The weight of these familial struggles undoubtedly added layers of complexity to O'Sullivan's already demanding professional career. Further complicating matters, O'Sullivan found himself embroiled in controversy at the 1996 World Championships when he admitted to assaulting a press officer. To top it all off, O'Sullivan faced private battles with addiction to drugs and alcohol, along with ongoing battles with depression and anxiety. These challenges added even more strain to an already turbulent phase in his life, posing a serious threat to both his personal wellbeing and professional career.

In recent years, O'Sullivan has taken significant steps toward managing his demons. He has sought professional help, engaged in therapy and adopted a healthier lifestyle to help manage his mental wellness.

Snooker presents a fascinating perspective on mental health, as it demands an immense level of mental resilience from its players. When a player misses a shot, they must endure the consequences of that mistake, while their opponent capitalizes on the opportunity to score. This dynamic can intensify the pressure, especially considering the prolonged duration of matches. Frames often last for 30 to 45 minutes, and in events like the World Championship final, which is played over two days and spans the best of 35 frames, the pressure can feel suffocating. The relentless nature of the competition, combined with the solitary nature of the game, amplifies the internal challenges faced by snooker players.

Most fans of the sport likely have some awareness of the personal struggles Ronnie O'Sullivan faced, given his occasional outbursts in the media. O'Sullivan has never been one to shy away from expressing criticism, whether directed at himself, his opponents or, often, the sport itself. However, it wasn't until recent behind-the-scenes footage surfaced from the 2022 World Championships final that the full extent of O'Sullivan's ongoing mental anguish became apparent.

O'Sullivan dominated day one of the final and raced into an early lead against his compatriot Judd Trump. However, on day two, as Trump mounted a comeback, chipping away at O'Sullivan's lead, the pressure visibly intensified. Exhaustion etched across O'Sullivan's face, his muscles tensed, and his face whitened; he found himself teetering on the brink of a panic attack. In a moment of raw vulnerability, he confessed, "On every shot, I think I'm going to miss... I'm scared."[58] This footage laid bare the psychological toll of high-stakes competition, offering a glimpse into the inner turmoil O'Sullivan grapples with amid the relentless demands of being the very best.

Despite the distressing scene, O'Sullivan somehow found the strength to compose himself and ultimately emerge victorious. However, the toll that even triumph takes on him is strikingly evident. In the footage, as he embraces Judd Trump in the aftermath, a microphone captures a confession in his moment of glory. O'Sullivan says to himself, "I can't do this anymore, I can't do it, it'll kill me."[59] Overwhelmed, he then buries his face in his teenage son's shoulder, tears streaming down his face uncontrollably.

This was the moment when O'Sullivan had just won his record-equalling seventh World Championship. Yet, he resembled a broken man. Years of relentless practice, fierce competition, and sky-high expectations converged, crashing down upon him in this moment. Despite the glory of victory, the toll of a lifetime devoted to snooker was evident.

In this snapshot of triumph tinged with melancholy, we could see the complexities of O'Sullivan's journey – a journey filled with remarkable success, but also shadowed by inner struggles and external pressures. Even in moments of triumph, the almost unparalleled pressure of professional sport can be suffocating.

PRESSURE AND PERFORMANCE – THRIVING IN FEARLESSNESS

The constant pressure experienced by athletes is associated with increased feelings of anxiety, and has even been shown to lead to a higher risk of injury.[60] Behind the scenes, athletes often endure a relentless battle with stress and pressure that can take a toll on their mental wellbeing. Recent research suggests that the demanding nature of elite sports can prompt an array of stressors, potentially triggering common mental disorders.[61]

Dr Pippa Grange is a renowned sports psychologist who has worked with countless world-class teams and organizations, including New Zealand Rugby, the Australian Olympic team and the English Football Association. Her groundbreaking work in the field of sports psychology has revolutionized the way we understand and approach mental wellbeing in high-pressure and competitive environments.

With a wealth of knowledge and expertise, Dr Grange has dedicated her career to helping athletes unlock their full potential. She does so by strengthening their mental resilience, enhancing their performance and nurturing their overall wellbeing. Her unique approach to psychological support goes beyond traditional methods, incorporating elements of empathy, authenticity and compassion that resonate deeply with those she works with.

In her innovative book *Fear Less*, Dr Grange asserts that there are two types of fear. The first is the type of fear you cannot fail to recognize, the panicky kind you feel before a job interview or a big speech. She refers to this as "in-the-moment fear".

The second type is "the kind that is running your life, making your choices and leaving you unfulfilled". She calls this the "not good enough fear". This is when emotions get mixed up with dread about what has happened in the past and what may happen in the future, and the fear of disappointing others or failing.[62] I'm certain it's a feeling that almost everyone can relate to. It's precisely the fear that discouraged me from embarking on the journey of writing this book for several years.

The culture of a sporting institution can play a pivotal role in triggering a fear of failure and the resulting mental health issues that often accompany it. In some "traditional" sporting cultures, we can observe cut-throat environments that prioritize winning at all costs. These environments foster the belief that fear and control are essential for driving performance.

However, it's worth considering, and even challenging, if this kind of fear-led environment is the best way of getting optimum performance from athletes. When sportspeople are constantly living in a heightened state of anxiety, it creates an atmosphere where the fear of failure and the consequences of poor performance feed into a vicious cycle. A classic example of this is the England cricket team of the 1990s. Despite boasting a highly talented squad, the environment around the team was ruthless – players were dropped and replaced for even a short period of poor form. As you can imagine, uncertainty and instability did not get the best out of this generation of players. This came to a head in 1999, when England hit rock bottom of the ICC test ranking for the first time, after losing a home series to New Zealand.[63]

This nadir led to a sweeping cultural change throughout English cricket, including the introduction of central contracts. And thus began a new era of cricket, where the most talented players were provided with greater assurances that they would maintain their place in the team through greater consistency in selection. This simple act of belief gave players the resilience to overcome rough patches and rediscover their top form. In just six years, the England team, including Marcus Trescothick, triumphed over a formidable Australian team, often hailed as the greatest in cricket history.

Turning a struggling team at the bottom of the world rankings into a powerhouse doesn't happen overnight. It is also not solely down to culture, but without providing high-quality players with the right environment, it will be nearly impossible for them to flourish. With the outcome-based nature of sport, there will always be pressure, but the best leaders are increasingly looking at ways to mitigate this and remove as many unnecessary stressors as possible to get the very best out of their players. We acknowledge the right societal environment is crucial to lay the foundations for the mental health revolution – the exact same principle can be applied to creating environments that allow athletes to flourish in the first place. Thankfully, voices like Dr Grange's are increasingly common and respected in the world of elite sport. This, I believe, is a crucial factor in creating an army of elite athletes who are leading the charge of the mental health revolution. As they become increasingly used to concepts such as vulnerability and fearlessness, the chances of them opening up publicly about their mental wellness will increase significantly.

NAVIGATING STRESS

The stress of competition can cast a shadow over much of an athlete's life, whether it be before, during or immediately after an event. This pressure is not limited solely to the moments of competition. It can seep into every aspect of a sportsperson's life, training, rehab, team meetings and even contract negotiations. The impact of stress on professional athletes cannot be overlooked. The pursuit of sporting excellence, combined with the expectations of fans, sponsors and team management, places a significant burden on these individuals.

Despite their seemingly glamorous lifestyle, professional sportspeople are not immune to pressure-related stress. As England cricket legend and mental health advocate Ben Stokes said recently, "It is a lot harder than it used to be. The more cricket that is played, the better for the sport, but you want a product that is of the highest quality... We are not cars where you can fill us up with petrol and let us go."[64]

Stokes perfectly illustrates why coaches and sport governing bodies need to be more in tune with their players' lives than ever before. Stokes is a cricketer of the very highest calibre and character. In 2019 alone, he produced two of the most remarkable innings ever played, just weeks apart, during the World Cup final and the Headingley Ashes test. Both innings were played under the most excruciating pressure, and on both occasions Stokes almost singlehandedly dragged his team to victory.

Judging solely by his sporting achievements, Ben Stokes might be the least likely candidate for needing support when it comes to handling pressure. His demeanour exudes confidence – he seemingly has nerves of steel and unwavering self-assurance in his skill and decision-making. He is a giant of the game.

Yet, in 2021 Stokes needed to take a six-month break from cricket after suffering a series of panic attacks. This was the culmination of a period when he was under extreme media scrutiny following his arrest and ultimate acquittal for an incident outside a Bristol nightclub. He was grieving the loss of his father who had just died. And all of this happened while the world lived in pandemic-enforced bio-bubbles, and cricketers continued to play around the world in front of empty stadiums.

There was significant pressure on the coffers of the England Cricket Board (ECB) to press ahead with matches during the Covid-19 pandemic. In fact, the meeting between England and the West Indies was the first international sporting event anywhere in the world during the pandemic.[65] However, the impact this period would have on players' and coaches' mental health was seemingly not factored into the equation. When not on the field, players lived alone in isolation for weeks on end, far away from their loved ones.

It is crucial for coaches and sporting bodies to recognize that athletes' lives extend beyond the field. There is a duty of care to protect them from the stresses that they may also be experiencing in their personal lives. The pandemic offered an extreme example of this, but even outside of times of global turmoil, it's important to know how athletes are *really* doing.

Thankfully, Dr Pippa Grange agrees that attitudes seem to be changing. She said, "Right now, there's a turning point in sport. You'll have seen evidence: the old school, predatory, possessive, controlling, fear-generating ways are finally being challenged."[66] Look at the example of the England cricket team: when the fear of losing their place was reduced, the players – and therefore the team – flourished.

Another potent example is the England national football team, with whom Dr Grange worked. In the 2000s and

2010s, England had a star-studded selection of players to choose from, to the extent that the team was dubbed the "golden generation". At club level, the players consistently challenged for and won the biggest prizes in football. Yet, when it came to the national team they failed. Fabio Capello, England's coach at the 2010 World Cup, was an archetypal old-school leader who created a culture of fear. Former England goalkeeper Joe Hart revealed the extent of the toxic atmosphere in the camp: "He was an extreme that none of us had experienced before. People were petrified of him... At best he called you by your surname. At worst you could tell in his head he was thinking, 'I don't know who you are.'"[67]

Compare this with the famously open, supportive and fearless environment fostered under the leadership of Gareth Southgate and Dr Pippa Grange. The team have flourished, reaching the semi-final of the World Cup in 2018 and the final of the Euro 2020, played in 2021. Some may even argue that the team achieved all this with a group of players that were inferior to Capello's during his fruitless era. Moreover, Southgate's squad made it to the top with an openness, honesty and integrity that has won them countless admirers in the process. And all of this stemmed from a coach in a role dubbed "the impossible job".[68]

Bringing about change requires a collective effort beyond the individual level to better support athletes' mental wellness. Changing the culture in a team or environment is never easy. It is something that takes vision, strategy, time and buy-in from all involved. It is something that can only really be achieved in a culture that values athletes' wellbeing alongside performance. However, when it is harnessed alongside world-class talent, the potential outcome is stratospheric.

Creating an atmosphere that is not driven by fear and judgement will not only aid performance. These environments are also much more likely to produce humans who are kind, empathetic and understanding – exactly the traits required in a generation of mental health advocates no longer shackled by the traditional views that have permeated sport and society for too long.

GREEN SHOOTS OF CHANGE

Thankfully, we are starting to see a trend of positive change amongst many high-profile athletes in the management of their own mental health. More athletes are taking that brave step, normalizing taking mental health breaks and prioritizing their own wellbeing.

A recent example of this is tennis player Naomi Osaka. The four-time Grand Slam winner made the difficult decision to withdraw from Roland Garros (also known as the French Open) in 2021. This move came just a day after Osaka was fined $15,000 by the French Open for refusing to engage with the press during the competition. She had expressed her intention to skip media obligations, citing the detrimental impact of these interactions on her mental wellbeing.

Osaka's decision to prioritize her mental health triggered debates about the treatment of athletes and the pressures they face in the media spotlight. Critics argue that the French Open's response, including the fine and the possibility of expulsion, were disproportionate, essentially forcing Osaka into a difficult choice between protecting her career or her mental health.

The withdrawal led to Osaka opening up about her long-standing battle with depression. She revealed that she had experienced bouts since the 2018 US Open final, where she defeated Serena Williams to claim her first Grand Slam title. This naturally led to significantly greater media attention, which intensified her struggles. On top of that, Osaka has described herself as an introverted individual who often wears headphones to help cope with social anxiety. She shared that she experiences immense nervousness before engaging with the media, making her decision to prioritize self-care and skip the press conferences in Paris completely understandable.[69]

Some athletes seem to have a natural gift when it comes to media duties. However, it stands to reason that not everyone will possess this skill set. It is, after all, very different to sporting talent. Some athletes who feel at home performing on the field or court can find answering questions from a room full of journalists a painful experience. Yet, fans increasingly want access to everything that surrounds sport: the build-up, the post-match analysis, the behind-the-scenes social media content.

Some argue that it's important for Naomi Osaka to toughen up and face activities she doesn't enjoy. They may say that this is just part of the deal of being a modern athlete. In recent years, resilience has taken centre stage as a buzzword in the realm of modern wellness.

Resilience has been heralded as a crucial attribute for navigating life's challenges and setbacks, fostering a sense of personal strength and adaptability. In a world marked by rapid changes, demanding work environments and personal struggles, being resilient is increasingly highly valued and seen as a sign of mental toughness. I know that I have personally put myself under immense pressure to be more resilient.

Yet, beneath the surface of this praise for resilience, there's a complex discussion about its potential harm when pushed too far, sometimes referred to as "toxic resilience". In fact, distinguishing between the promotion of wellness-driven resilience and the old-school attitudes of past generations isn't easy. Upon closer examination, they seem quite alike to me.

While resilience undoubtedly plays a role in helping individuals cope with stressors and emerge stronger, the belief that one must constantly display unwavering resilience can surely only lead to burnout and detrimental outcomes. It also creates harmful expectations that individuals should effortlessly overcome every obstacle and maintain a facade of invincibility. The pressure to consistently demonstrate resilience is unrealistic and can only end in failure.

It's also possible that the emphasis on excessive resilience may inadvertently discourage people from seeking help when needed. It can create a culture that stigmatizes seeking support, as individuals may fear being perceived as weak or incapable if they admit to struggling. This is the exact opposite of the functioning environment that elite sports should be fostering.

It is essential to strike a balance between promoting resilience and recognizing the value of vulnerability. For this reason, I celebrate the self-compassion that Naomi Osaka displayed in choosing her wellness ahead of a tennis tournament, no matter how prestigious.

Media rights are a huge source of income for events such as the French Open, and broadcasters are demanding more content than ever before. However, in this new and evolving media landscape, it is up to all parties involved to recognize when talent needs protection – when enough is enough. Surely no one is happy when one of the biggest names in the sport withdraws from a marquee event. When any athlete must choose between their careers and their mental health, then we have gone too far in our demands. We shouldn't be asking athletes to show more resilience – we should ask ourselves how much of their time, energy and focus is enough.

FROM MASTERY TO NOVICE – THE VANISHING ACT

If we expect athletes to take a leading role in the mental health revolution, we must also reflect on our own interactions with them. If we don't actively contribute, it will hinder progress or even disrupt the process entirely. One crucial step is to consider how we, as fans, respond to athletes during their lowest points in their professional careers.

When I was growing up, sportspeople who struggled with pressure to perform were euphemistically labelled as "mentally weak". The struggle that comes with what can almost appear to be instantaneous loss of form has also been referred to as "the yips" or "choking".

The yips have always captivated psychologists, coaches and sports fans alike because of their mysterious nature. Across the history of sports, numerous top athletes have been affected by the yips, experiencing a sudden and notable decline in performance that seems to come out of nowhere.

Chuck Knoblauch, a once-promising baseball player, famously fell victim to the yips. Knoblauch emerged as a highly talented second baseman, with exceptional defensive skills and a solid batting average. The early stages of his career showcased a player destined for greatness. Knoblauch was already a four-time All-Star and a World Series champion with the Minnesota Twins when he was traded to the biggest team in Major League Baseball, the New York Yankees.

Once on the team, Knoblauch developed significant issues performing the most basic skill of a second baseman: throwing the ball to first base. Knoblauch committed 26 errors during the 1999 campaign. It got worse still by the time the Yankees played the White Sox in June 2000. Knoblauch committed three errors in just six innings before taking himself out of the game. Two days later, he fired a throw so wide of the mark that it hit broadcaster Keith Olbermann's mother in the Yankee Stadium seats.

As Knoblauch's woes continued to escalate, the media scrutiny intensified. His struggle became a magnet for media attention. Reporters and journalists fixated on his declining performance, magnifying every error and dissecting his struggles in minute detail, amplifying the torment of an athlete already besieged by his own internal demons.

The thing that sets the yips apart from other serious psychological challenges that athletes may face is the kind of peculiar glee it seems to elicit from outsiders. When Knoblauch threw the ball that hit Keith Olbermann's mother, the commentators laughed and joked about how she had probably just lost a filling. However, in reality, what we were witnessing was an athlete so low on confidence that an action that had been honed and perfected over a lifetime of practice had simply evaporated. That person needs sympathy, not ridicule.

THE WORST OVER OF ALL TIME

Another player who was severely affected by performance pressure was Scott Boswell. At the age of 26, Boswell was a seasoned cricketer, enjoying a successful career at Leicestershire. He had become a regular in their one-day side and was in prime form during the season leading up to the Cheltenham & Gloucester Trophy final. The team was on a winning streak, and, in part due to Boswell's outstanding performance in the semi, secured their spot in the final against Somerset. It was by far the biggest game of his career to date.

However, that day turned into a nightmare that would haunt Boswell for years to come. Many cricket fans will have seen the infamous video titled "The Worst Over Ever?" on YouTube that circulates every so often. The video showcases Boswell's struggle as he bowled six wides in his first eight balls, with five consecutive wides at one point. The opposing batsman, Marcus Trescothick (remember him?), capitalized on the erratic deliveries, hitting a couple of straighter balls for four.

That disastrous over marked the end of Boswell's professional cricket career. The events of that day left a lasting impact on his life, Boswell himself admitted that it took him around ten years to come to terms with the events of that day.

The night before the final, Boswell had been struggling with his form. The coaches were uncertain about his selection, and a senior figure at the club told him bluntly "not to fuck up", a classic move in a fear-led environment. Those words stayed with him, adding to the mounting pressure. When it came time for him to bowl, his nerves got the better of him. As he bowled to Trescothick in his second over, his vision became distorted, and panic set in. He lost control, bowling a series of wides as the crowd's roar grew louder. His muscles tightened, his fingers clenched and sweat formed on his brow. The more he panicked, the worse it got.

Throughout this ordeal, no one spoke to him. He wanted it to be over, but it seemed never-ending. The umpire urged him to keep bowling, and Boswell's fear intensified. He was terrified that the over would continue indefinitely.[70] Finally, the over concluded at the expense of 23 runs. Boswell's embarrassment reached its peak when he missed a catch and tore up a chunk of the Lord's turf. Frozen on the field, he couldn't even walk a few yards to fetch a water bottle.

The aftermath of the match was equally devastating. Boswell's teammates and the cricketing community distanced themselves from him. Leicestershire terminated his contract, effectively bringing an end to his career as a professional sportsman.

The yips and pressure to perform present a perplexing challenge. Far too often the yips have been trivialized. However, the impact of this condition can have long-lasting consequences on the sufferer. Imagine not being able to execute a basic skill in your day job, one that you'd performed perfectly countless times before. Think about the consequences that would have on your mental wellbeing, capacity to earn money and general sense of worth. Now, imagine that incident being filmed for prosperity and being shared across the internet. The sheer number of clips online that rubberneck the very worst moments of athletes' careers reveal how much enjoyment we take in the failure of elite sportspeople. This is particularly true when said athletes represent a rival team.

There is no doubt a degree of schadenfreude that can be taken from sportspeople failing, particularly in the case of the yips, when they seem to be unable to execute the most basic requirements of their sport. Witnessing an athlete fail can evoke a sense of satisfaction in some. Perhaps this provides a brief reprieve from their own challenges or insecurities. It may serve as a subconscious reminder that even those we idolize are not exempt from the trials and tribulations of life.

The fascination with witnessing athletes fail is a complex aspect of human nature. When someone is living out a personal and professional nightmare in front of a television audience, we really should examine any joy we feel in that. Personally, I believe we ought to rise above such impulses. During a moment of envy toward a colleague's accomplishments, a mentor once reminded me, "Success isn't a limited commodity." It's crucial to acknowledge that embracing others' successes ultimately enriches our own sense of fulfilment.

WHERE DO THE YIPS COME FROM?

So, why does this happen? Why do skills that have been honed over years of practice suddenly evaporate?

As with all motor skill-based activities, we progress from a developmental stage to mastery. Whether it's learning to walk or sinking a 15-foot putt, we inevitably experience an awkward transition phase, during which we acquire the optimal muscle movements required to perform each task.

Russell Poldrack, a neuroscientist at the University of California, conducted a series of experiments that tracked brain activity at different stages of skill mastery. He discovered that the prefrontal cortex is activated when a novice is learning, but over time, as the skill becomes more well-known and honed, it switches to a completely different part of the brain, the basal ganglia. Although we are in essence doing the same activity, the part of the brain that we use to execute it varies depending on the level of mastery we have over any specific task.[71]

A frequently cited example of this is the process we go through when learning to drive. Anyone who has done this knows the first few times behind a wheel are stressful experiences. I remember feeling drained after each of my early driving lessons, due to the sheer mental energy exerted. Every gear change, every indicator signal, every parking manoeuvre requires your undivided attention. Then, before you know it, you can effortlessly execute a series of complex manoeuvres with ease, while holding a conversation with your passengers. So, applying what Poldrack and the team at the University of California found, during the early phase of this process, you are using your prefrontal cortex. By the time you become a skilled driver, you are tapping into your honed abilities in the basal ganglia.

Now, let's think about this in terms of the complex skills that athletes regularly execute. If you asked Formula One driver Lewis Hamilton to describe the symphony of movements he goes through as he approaches a corner at 120mph, or tennis player Coco Gauff what she does with her feet or hips to generate extra whip on a forehand, they would not be able to adequately explain it – at least not at an accurate biomechanical level. This is because so much of the process is deeply embedded in the basal ganglia and executed almost subconsciously.

This is perhaps one of the primary reasons why being a great player does not always translate to being a great coach. Although many outstanding players transition into exceptional coaches, their success is likely down to their exposure to world-class trainers and their capacity to absorb and apply knowledge, rather than their athletic abilities. This distinction is crucial, due to the vast differences between excelling as an athlete and understanding the intricacies of skill execution in sports, particularly in how our brains process these skills.

So, let's return to those individuals experiencing the yips, or choking, or however we wish to characterize it. It appears that the most plausible explanation lies in moments of intense stress. For instance, during the most significant game of Scott Boswell's career, or following Knoblauch's trade to the most famous franchise in baseball, the desire for success became so overwhelming and incapacitating that they ceased to rely on their finely tuned skills. They stopped tapping into the basal ganglia, which would normally guide them through these moments with relative ease. They started thinking about their skills and their actions. If anything, they were trying too hard.

This is the lethal breeding ground of the yips, because the more you think about the minutiae of each process, your brain switches back to the learning phase – the prefrontal cortex takes over. This explains why Knoblauch, a four-time All-Star and World Series champion, looked like a rank amateur. It explains why he was unable to execute a skill that you would expect a decent high-school player to nail. It's all the fault of the prefrontal cortex.

Think of it in the following way: if someone asked you to walk ten yards in a straight line, staying within a boundary of ten inches on each side, I would guess that the completion rate of such a task amongst able-bodied people would be close to 100 per cent. Now, imagine being asked to walk ten yards across a half-yard-wide beam, suspended high in the air. On the surface, it is exactly the same task. It requires the same basic skill set to execute, and yet the variable of being suspended high in the air transforms it into something entirely new. This newness forces the prefrontal cortex to take over. Even if we manage to complete the task, it's highly likely that we would do so with uncertain footing and less finesse compared to when we're on solid ground.

Understanding the neuroscience behind the yips is helpful in a couple of ways. Firstly, by gaining a deeper understanding of the mechanics behind the yips, it gives athletes and coaches a fighting chance to counter them when they surface. It allows a certain amount of forward planning by developing strategies that may give athletes a chance to switch back to the basal ganglia, where automatic performance is rooted.

Additionally, from the perspective of this book's aim to highlight the important role that athletes can play in the mental health revolution, the very existence of choking or the yips helps to demonstrate that athletes are not robots or superhuman. The skills they possess are not locked in for life. With the wrong combination of triggers, even the most skilled athletes can succumb to a sudden, extreme loss of form, all caused by the wrong part of their brain taking over. Perhaps control of this aspect is what separates the best from the rest. As former six-time world snooker champion Steve Davis suggests, you need to learn the art of "playing as if it means nothing, when it means everything".[72]

THE SPOTLIGHT – CAN YOU HANDLE THE GLARE?

When we think of elite athletes, we often picture them basking in the glory of their achievements, adored by fans and celebrated by the media. However, behind the scenes, there is often a lesser-known reality: some sportspeople grapple with the overwhelming weight of fame.

While fame may seem glamorous, it can take a toll on an athlete's mental health. For truly world-class athletes in highly visible sports, fame is an inevitable side-effect of their profession, whether they like it or not. And being in the public eye comes with an incessant demand for attention, constant scrutiny and an invasion of personal privacy. Athletes are expected to perform not only on the field but also off it, becoming ambassadors for their sport and role models for their fans. However, not all athletes are comfortable with the pressures and expectations that come with fame.

Loss of privacy can be particularly challenging for athletes who prefer a quiet life. Constant media attention, paparazzi and public scrutiny can leave them feeling exposed and vulnerable. Fame is not a tap that you can turn on and off. Even mundane activities, like shopping or going out for a meal with your family, become significant logistical missions when you are a well-known celebrity. This is particularly true in the age of the smartphone. Every person you encounter is armed with a camera, and any lapse in behaviour is likely to go viral within minutes.

Additionally, unlike many other drivers of celebrity, such as acting, politics or even reality television, sport is largely non-verbal. Therefore, it would stand to reason that you would naturally expect to see a greater proportion of introverts in sport than within those other disciplines. Perhaps this is the same reason why, among musicians, the lead singer tends to lap up the limelight more than other members of the band, who are happy to hide behind their instruments. Naomi Osaka illustrates this point perfectly. Despite her discomfort in front of the press pack, it has no bearing on her exceptional skills as a tennis player. There seem to be a number of athletes that long for the days when they could go about their lives without attracting quite so much attention, or having every move analysed.

Elite athletes are also expected to maintain an image in the public eye that portrays confidence and invincibility. However, like us, they are human beings who experience emotions and struggles. The pressure to constantly perform and live up to expectations can lead to feelings of anxiety, self-doubt and fear of failure. The thought of letting down fans and teammates can be a heavy burden to bear. As mentioned, this is only amplified when any mistakes are made, not only on the field of play, but also in real life.

Rightly or wrongly, there is a societal expectation that sportspeople should be role models. This is driven by the superhero status that many young people reserve for athletes. While I think most athletes do an admirable job fulfilling this role, and serve as wonderful role models for children, I also believe that it's not inherently tied to their profession. If athletes opt out of being seen as role models to alleviate the extra pressure it brings, I completely respect their decision to do so.

Paradoxically, the fame that comes with being an elite athlete can also lead to feelings of isolation and loneliness. The hectic schedules, constant travel and time away from loved ones can leave athletes feeling disconnected from their support systems. A prime example of this is the way that Ben Stokes struggled with being separated from his family during the height of the Covid-19 pandemic, as discussed earlier in this chapter. The consequences of the lack of a proper support system on an athlete's mental wellbeing can have devastating consequences. In the Stokes example, it led to him being out of the sport for a comparable time as a serious physical injury would have incurred. This should raise serious alarm bells to all coaches and administrators about the consequences of not valuing the mental wellbeing of athletes.

THE BURDEN OF BRIGHT LIGHTS – DERRICK ROSE'S RELATIONSHIP WITH FAME

Derrick Rose is a professional basketball player, who has played for the Chicago Bulls, New York Knicks and Memphis Grizzlies, among others. He is known for his introverted nature and his antipathy to fame. Throughout his career, Rose has faced numerous challenges, both personal and professional, that have put his mental health under strain. From early success to recurring injuries and media scrutiny, Rose never really adjusted to the glare of the media.

Despite his numerous accomplishments and skills that allowed him to rise to the top of his profession, Rose has always been uncomfortable with the fame that comes with being a professional athlete. He acknowledges the blessings of his position but admits that he despises the spotlight. He has said, "I picked the profession I'm in, so there's no way I could whine about it. And I'm blessed enough to be in this position... but I hate fame. It's just not who I am."[73]

Rose's journey began with controversy during his college years, when allegations of academic misconduct tarnished his achievements. Moving on to the National Basketball Association (NBA), injuries became a constant hurdle, hampering his performance and disappointing fans. These setbacks, combined with off-court controversies, have contributed to a mixed perception of Rose and fuelled criticism from the media and fans alike.

Rose's introverted nature and reluctance to conform to media expectations have often been misinterpreted as a lack of intelligence or media savviness. The criticism he has faced is tinged with racial undertones. As an individual who prefers solitude, Rose has struggled to find a balance between staying true to himself and meeting the demands of public perception.

As previously mentioned, injuries have played a significant role in Rose's career, causing physical pain and emotional distress. The documentary *The Return* provided fans with a glimpse into the inner turmoil Rose experienced after tearing his ACL (anterior cruciate ligament), highlighting the toll it took on his mental wellbeing.

Similarly, Rose's upbringing in Chicago's violence-plagued Englewood neighbourhood shaped his character and instilled a strong work ethic. However, it also made him hesitant to open up and seek help when facing personal challenges.

Rose's critics often view him through a narrow lens, failing to understand his introverted nature and the nuances of his personality. His desire for privacy and reluctance to conform to media expectations have created a divide between him and the public. However, despite the criticism, Rose maintains a dedicated fan base, particularly in his hometown of Chicago, where he remains an inspirational figure for many.

ARE WE GETTING THE MOST OUT OF ATHLETES?

There is an expectation that fame is part of the deal when someone becomes a star athlete. Yet, in the same way we should not expect sportspeople to be natural media darlings, why would we expect them to love fame? From Derrick Rose to Naomi Osaka to, in my opinion, the greatest footballer of all time, Lionel "Leo" Messi, sport is littered with stars who seem to have little interest in being famous.

By constantly forcing professional athletes to supplement their finite time and energy with media and sponsorship commitments, we surely are not getting the best out of them. I understand the economics of sport means that the lavish wages that elite athletes earn would not be possible without media commitments. Yet, I would prefer to live in a utopian world where athletes are free to maximize their talents.

As absurd as they may sound, I'd like to pose a few questions. Did we get the most out of Leo Messi's career? What if the mechanics of modern football had somehow allowed him to concentrate solely on his game? As unfathomable as it may seem, in perfect conditions, could Messi have been even better?

In the great book *Flow* by Mihaly Csikszentmihalyi, he theorizes that optimal performance is only possible when the skills possessed are balanced to the challenge and external distractions are minimized. This state is referred to as "flow". He describes the characteristics of flow as a state of "concentration that is so intense that there is no attention left over to think about anything irrelevant. Self-consciousness disappears and the sense of time is distorted."[74] Any sports fan will know from post-match interviews that elite athletes sometimes refer to this state as "being in the zone". Those who compete in fast-moving team sports – football, hockey or American football, for example – may say that time seems to slow down. Batters in cricket or baseball often say the ball seems bigger and easier to hit, while basketball players may feel like the hoop is larger than normal. What all these athletes have in common is that they have reached a state of flow.

Csikszentmihalyi argues that sport is inherently structured to encourage athletes to enter flow states. They are structured realities that are based on the foundations of repeatable skills. Even the ritual of dressing up in team uniforms and entering a special arena for competition is advantageous in terms of reaching flow. And yet, having listened to several elite athletes talk on the subject, the state of true flow can be fleeting. It's not like a tap that can be turned on and off. I have heard many elite sportspeople say that they only felt truly "in the zone" a handful of times in their careers.

In order to reach a flow state more often, Csikszentmihalyi suggests that athletes primarily focus on the activity, rather than the surrounding noise that comes with being a star player. If extrinsic goals, such as beating your opponent, wanting to impress the audience or signing a new contract, are of greater importance, you are less likely to ascend to flow than if you primarily focus on the activity itself. This is perhaps why, after a particularly good performance, so many elite athletes say that it felt like they were a child again, playing with their friends, just for the love of the game.

According to Csikszentmihalyi, that is the key to unlocking the state of flow – and that is where the magic happens.

Based on this, we must ask: do sport administrators have a duty to provide the best possible conditions for each athlete to flourish, or must they simply create an environment that maximizes revenues? Should we as fans demand that athletes are given a platform for optimal performance? Do we really need to see another tedious interview with a sportsperson who is media trained to within an inch of their lives? Looking at the specific example of Leo Messi, perhaps he is just supernaturally good at tapping into that state of flow. Perhaps he has an ability to quieten all the external noise and play for the sheer joy of the game. However, the opposite may also be true, and his ceiling of potential may have been even higher. We may just be talking about a percentage point or two, but if you offered me the chance to see yet another dull interview or a 1–2 per cent uplift in his on-field performance, I know which one I would choose.

Part of the reason why I wanted to acknowledge this group of athletes who detest fame is because I want to highlight the diversity of personalities among professional athletes. No matter how much progress we collectively make in the mental health revolution, it stands to reason that some will always feel uncomfortable with their status as the poster child for any cause. That is absolutely fine. Expecting anything else would only make me a hypocrite. Yet, if we go back to the incredible statistic that nearly 42 per cent of the Canadian Olympic team suffered from a diagnosable mental condition, then surely a mental health revolution could be spearheaded by the extroverts. For the more introverted athletes, well, they can just focus on their game and hopefully ascend to a state of flow as frequently as possible, while their outspoken teammates lead the charge.

MODERN PRESSURES

In modern times, another form of pressure has emerged. It's something that impacts most of us, and elite athletes are no different. We now live in a world where social media dominates our lives, creating a sense of pressure to always be "on", always be connected and always be achieving. Young people are growing up in an environment where their worth is measured by the number of likes, followers and shares they get, rather than by their accomplishments or character.

Sports stars are no strangers to the spotlight – everything they do seems to be scrutinized by fans and journalists alike. In recent years, social media has become a crucial tool for athletes to connect with their audiences, and many have embraced it with open arms. From sharing behind-the-scenes glimpses into their lives, to engaging with fans in real time, sportspeople are using social media in increasingly creative ways.

Take footballer Cristiano Ronaldo, for example. At the time of writing this book, the Portuguese superstar is the most followed person on Instagram, with more than 600 million followers. He regularly posts pictures and videos of himself training, relaxing with his family and promoting his various business ventures. But it's not just about self-promotion – Ronaldo also uses his platform to highlight important social causes, such as the fight against racism.

Another footballer who has harnessed social media is Marcus Rashford. The English footballer has become a vocal advocate for social justice, using his platform to campaign for better school meals for children and highlight the issue of child poverty. Rashford's activism has earned him widespread praise and admiration, and he has even been awarded an MBE for his services to charity.

It's not just footballers who are using social media to make a difference. American basketball star LeBron James has been an advocate for racial equality, using his platform to call for justice for victims of police brutality and support for the Black Lives Matter movement. Meanwhile, tennis legend Serena Williams has used social media to promote gender equality and highlight the struggles faced by working mothers.

Regardless of how they use their social platforms, there's no denying that social media has become an essential tool for sports stars. It allows them to connect with fans on a more personal level, promote their brands and business ventures, and share their views and opinions with the world. Of course, with social media always evolving and changing, it's hard to say how they will continue to use it in the future.

It also underlines the point that sports stars are incredibly influential in a decentralized media landscape. The two most followed individuals on Instagram are both footballers: Ronaldo and Messi. The rest of the top 50 most popular accounts includes wrestlers, cricketers, basketball players and, yes, a smattering of other footballers. We live in an era where individual sports stars have never had more direct influence. As outlined above, they are also no strangers at using their platforms for good, which is precisely why I believe they are such an important component in the mental health revolution.

REVOLUTION OR DISTRACTION

Conversely, in the rarefied air of elite sports, you may wonder if social media is an unnecessary distraction. If Ronaldo didn't have 600 million Instagram followers, would his profile or bank balance be noticeably diminished?

One of the biggest issues with social media for sportspeople is the potential for it to be a time-consuming distraction. With constant notifications, messages and updates, athletes can easily lose focus on their training and competition preparation.

If we take the concept of marginal gains, made famous by cycling coach Sir Dave Brailsford, social media could easily be seen as something that could diminish performance. Brailsford's philosophy stems from the belief that achieving substantial progress does not always require radical changes, but rather a collection of small improvements that accumulate over time. Instead of focusing solely on major breakthroughs, Brailsford's approach involves examining every aspect of an athlete's performance and seeking marginal improvements in each area. This method extends beyond physical training and delves into areas such as equipment, nutrition, recovery, mindset and even personal hygiene.

To put the marginal gains theory into practice, Brailsford took a systematic approach within the British Cycling team. He encouraged riders, coaches and staff to question everything and experiment with novel strategies. Some of the areas where marginal gains were sought included bike frame design, tire pressure, nutrition plans, sleep optimization, clothing aerodynamics and hand-washing techniques to reduce illness.

The marginal gains theory proved to be a game-changer for British Cycling. Under Brailsford's leadership from 1997 to 2014, the British Cycling team achieved unprecedented success at the Olympic Games and Tour de France. The team's domination in the sport can be attributed, at least in part, to the relentless pursuit of marginal improvements across every aspect of performance. Brailsford's philosophy has since been adopted by other sports teams and organizations worldwide, revolutionizing their approach to training and performance optimization.[75]

When we look at social media through the filter of the marginal gains philosophy, it's not hard to see how it could become a distraction that could lead to a decrease in performance. At the very elite level of competition, athletes can't afford to give away any advantage, given the incredibly fine margins between victory and defeat.

Another issue with social media is the potential for it to be a source of negativity and criticism. Elite sportspeople are often in the public eye, and this can make them a target for abuse and trolling. This can be especially harmful to their mental health and could also potentially impact their athletic performance.

Though social media is a relatively new phenomenon, the link between athletic performance and excessive usage is something that is already fairly well explored. The initial results do not look favourable.

Firstly, there was a review of NBA game statistics between 2009 and 2016 among more than 100 verified Twitter-using NBA players. It uncovered that those who were posting late at night, between the hours of 11pm and 7am, scored significantly fewer points and achieved fewer rebounds in games played the following day.[76]

During the Beijing Olympics in 2008, there were 100 million Facebook users globally; by the next games held in London in 2012, that number had swelled to more than 900 million.[77] This meant that the London games were the first where social media had truly cut through into the mainstream. This not only offered exciting new ways to follow the games, but it also had an impact on the athletes themselves.

An article published by the website Bleacher Report just before the London games on the training regimen of swimmer and three-time gold medallist in Beijing, Stephanie Rice, hinted at a newly formed addiction to social media. "With her focus on winning gold at the Olympics, Rice's social life is low-key. Most nights she is in bed by 10pm, distracted only by social media, replying to Twitter messages or checking Facebook," revealed the report.[78]

Then, at the London games, Rice placed fourth in one event and sixth in another, an underwhelming showing after she broke the World Record on the way to gold in the same two events in Beijing. Now, a swimmers' career is vanishingly short, so a performance drop-off over four years is not unusual. However, Rice was just 24 years old in London and injury-free, so many expected her to perform significantly better.

Fellow Australian swimmer and teammate of Rice, Emily Seebohm, was a favourite to win gold in her event, the 100-metre backstroke. However, she missed out by a fraction of a second to American Missy Franklin. Afterwards, she admitted to journalists that she had been spending an excessive amount of time online and that may have impacted her performance. She confessed that she "... didn't really get off social media".[79]

Motivated by the Rice and Seebohm incidents, Australian researchers embarked on a study to examine whether there might be a correlation between social media use and sport anxiety. This is a specific form of social anxiety that can impact athletic performance. It is believed to also play a role in the occurrence of sports injuries, rehabilitation and the timing of an athlete's return to sport.

To investigate any potential links between social media use and sport anxiety, the researchers enlisted the participation of nearly 300 athletes from 13 different countries. The participants were asked to rank themselves on the Sport

Anxiety Scale (SAS) and complete a questionnaire regarding their social media usage. The findings revealed that nearly one-third of the athletes checked social media during competitions, and more than two-thirds of users checked the platform at least two hours before competing. Interestingly, the researchers found that "the closer an athlete accessed social media to the start of the competition, the greater the disruption to their concentration".[80]

These findings should raise significant concerns for athletes and coaches alike. Social media has the potential to serve as a major distraction, impeding athletes' ability to psychologically prepare and maintain focus during competition. In the world of marginal gains, it appears that athletes should probably shun social media altogether, but particularly in the immediate build-up to an event.

This is especially concerning when you consider that most elite athletes tend to be young men and women. They are often working through many personal and developmental milestones in front of the general public, who can be unforgiving of mistakes. And, since the 2012 Olympics, we have seen ever greater penetration and proliferation of social media platforms. We now have a generation of young athletes who have grown up with social media as a normal part of their daily existence, so weaning themselves off these platforms, even just for a few hours at a time, is likely to prove challenging. Yet, the psychological benefits could help them reach a heightened level of performance, and be the difference between them being good and being great.

Social media has also been criticized for its relentless focus on appearance, leading to a rise in anxiety, depression and other mental health issues. New research is suggesting that this is disproportionately affecting female athletes. A study conducted by researchers at Rocky Vista University in Colorado has revealed that platforms like Instagram and Facebook have intensified the pressure on young women to achieve unrealistic body standards.[81] This pressure has led to distressing accounts of extreme measures taken by athletes to adhere to these "ideals".

The study highlights the role of fitness influencers, celebrities and fashion models in spreading false information and presenting photoshopped, unattainable body images. This phenomenon, commonly referred to as "fitspiration", is widespread across various social media platforms. Eating disorders among athletes, whether they're at the elite or developmental levels, are, unfortunately, widespread. Athletes, including Olympic gold medallist Jessie Diggins and former elite gymnast Vanessa Atler, have bravely shared their struggles with eating disorders.

To address this growing issue, medical experts Kathryn Vidlock, Catherine Liggett and Andrew Dole propose a comprehensive approach that includes providing healthy eating and nutrition guidance to young women at all levels of athletic participation. In their book, *Spring Forward: Balanced Eating, Exercise and Body Image in Sport for Female Athletes*, they outline potential solutions and have developed an education program for schools called SPRING, an acronym for Strength and Positivity Rooted in Nutrition for Girls. The program aims to increase body image "flexibility" and boost confidence in one's body, regardless of size or shape. Encouragingly, data from their research indicates a 22 per cent increase in body image flexibility among female athletes following the implementation of the program.[82]

Parents and coaches also play a crucial role in preventing eating disorders among young athletes. By promoting open communication, providing support and fostering a positive environment, parents and coaches can help athletes develop a healthy relationship with their bodies. Shifting the focus from appearance to performance and overall wellbeing can help build resilience against the pressures of social media.

Fortunately, online platforms are also helping combat the negative pressure that comes with social media. YouTube has updated its guidelines to address disordered eating. Now, they prohibit content that promotes behaviours that could be imitated by vulnerable individuals. This includes banning content showing restrictive eating, calorie restriction, purging and weight-based bullying.[83]

A KICK AGAINST MISOGYNY – TAYLA HARRIS AND THE BATTLE FOR RESPECT ONLINE

Female athletes continue to experience a significant amount of sexualization and judgement based on their looks. Sadly, there are far too many examples of this, but let's look at the case of Tayla Harris, which perfectly illustrates this ongoing problem.

Harris, an Australian rules footballer, found herself at the centre of a controversy in March 2019 when a photograph of her mid-kick went viral. If you haven't seen the image, I suggest you do a quick search for it online now. It captures her mid-air, kicking the ball away, demonstrating perfect technique with her kicking boot stretched high above her own head. It is an image that perfectly captures power, technique and athleticism honed over years of hard practice.

The image was initially shared by Channel 7, the Australian television network broadcasting the match. However, the photo quickly became a target for online trolls who posted sexist and derogatory comments, turning a celebratory moment into a platform for misogyny.[84]

Rather than succumbing to the harassment, Harris took a bold stand. She shared the photo on her own social media accounts, accompanied by a powerful message condemning the comments. She wrote, "Here's a pic of me at work... think about this before your derogatory comments."[85] Her response to the barrage of abuse she faced that day gained widespread support, not just from the sports community, but from people around the world who were appalled by the reaction to the image.

The Tayla Harris photo ignited a significant shift in public opinion, with many finally recognizing the urgent need to address the prevalent issue of online harassment faced by women. It highlighted the rampant sexism ingrained within sports and social media platforms. The incident became a rallying cry for change, sparking important conversations about gender equality, representation and the role of media in perpetuating harmful narratives.

It is clear that social media platforms have a responsibility to create and enforce policies that protect users from abusive behaviour. When it comes to social media, the genie is well and truly out of the bottle. For the majority of young people today, social media is a staple of their everyday lives and a key method of self-expression. As such, it is extremely important for other social media platforms to follow YouTube and implement stricter policies to protect users from harmful content that promotes unrealistic body standards, abuse and misogyny.

There are real-life consequences to online actions. According to one research study, victims of cyberbullying are twice as likely to experience suicidal thoughts and behaviours, as well as self-harm.[86] Social media's biggest platforms could and should be doing more to stop the truly ugly side of their business. This is a non-negotiable piece of progress that needs to be made, or we risk someone more vulnerable than Tayla Harris falling victim to online trolling and there being serious consequences.

As with almost any large technological leap forward, it takes some time to realize the consequences of the new tools. It is clear that social media can be harnessed for good. When we think about athletes spearheading the mental health revolution, social media is certainly one of the key weapons in the armoury of the movement, as it allows athletes to talk directly to their fans about key issues.

Yet, you don't need to scratch too far below the surface to reveal the corrosive elements of social media, which, if left unchecked, could prove to be a significant barrier to the mental health revolution. There is mounting evidence that social media has the power to potentially worsen athletic performance and diminish mental wellness. Therefore, despite its incredible power, it is something that must be used with great caution, particularly while platforms fail to acknowledge the duty of care they have for their users. As long as trolls, hatemongers and purveyors of harmful content are protected on these sites, there will always be a barrier that prevents athletes from opening up about their own mental health experiences. This is something we should not accept or tolerate from our fellow social media users or the platforms themselves.

6

WOMEN'S MENTAL HEALTH IN SPORT

Breaking Barriers

In recent years, women's sports have made significant strides in terms of mainstream recognition and popularity. What was once a niche market consigned to a handful of sports has become a vital part of the global sporting landscape, in the process attracting millions of viewers and fans worldwide. However, as the Tayla Harris incident discussed in the previous chapter demonstrates, we still have a long way to go before male and female athletes are treated equally.

One of the primary drivers behind the growing popularity of women's sports is simply down to increased visibility and representation. In the past, women's sports received little coverage in mainstream media, with the focus being on male competitors. Outside of the Olympics and Wimbledon fortnight, female athletes barely received any mainstream media coverage throughout my childhood in the UK. However, the tide has started to turn, with broadcasters and newspapers dedicating more airtime and column inches to women's sports than ever before.

It also appears there was a market there the whole time. A peak TV audience of more than 17 million people tuned in to watch England's historic win over Germany in the Women's Euro 2022 final. This made it not only the most-watched women's football game in UK television history, but also the most-watched TV event of the year, full stop.[87] This kind of audience for a women's football match in the UK would have been unimaginable 20 years ago, largely because it would not have had the exposure or promotion to push it to such heights.

Although there will always likely be a misogynistic group among football fans who belittle the women's game, it is heartening to note that most women's football fans are actually men.[88] It becomes evident that by continuously exposing and promoting the game, there is a possibility of reversing deep-seated attitudes.

It also stands to reason that the more high-profile athletes we have in the mainstream consciousness, the greater potential there is for more troops to join the mental health revolution. There is also a societal aspect at play here, as one could argue that women may be culturally more open to discussions related to mental health. Dr Pippa Grange points out that "repressing emotions is a culturally learned behaviour. It has been especially encouraged in boys and men, who have often been conditioned to believe that showing fear is a sign of weakness."[89] Therefore, having more high-profile female athletes may not only be a benefit for the mental health revolution, but it might also be a prerequisite.

SOCIAL MEDIA AND ACTIVISM

In the last chapter, we discussed the corrosive and harmful side of social media. However, I also recognize its immense power and potential. Numerous female athletes have used their social platforms as a way of reaching a wider global audience, bypassing traditional media gatekeepers and raising awareness of important issues in the process.

Social media has undeniably played a significant role in enhancing the visibility of women's sports. Female athletes, like their male counterparts, amass millions of followers on various social platforms. Interestingly, these platforms, which, as we've seen, can harbour misogynistic hate, also offer opportunities to promote greater gender equality in sports. They provide a means for athletes to speak out on important issues. A notable example in football is the US Women's National Team (USWNT), which has actively advocated for equal pay through social media.

The USWNT is widely recognized as one of the most successful football teams in history, having secured four World Cups and four Olympic gold medals since 1991. However, despite their remarkable achievements, the female players on the team have consistently received significantly lower compensation than their male counterparts. This glaring disparity came to light during the team's 2019 lawsuit against the United States Soccer Federation (USSF). It revealed that male players were being paid more, despite the fact that the women's team generated higher revenue for the USSF. According to court documents, female players were paid just 38 cents for every dollar earned by the men.[90]

The USWNT's fight for equal pay has been met with support from fans, politicians and fellow athletes. In 2020, the team received an outpouring of support on International Women's Day, with people around the world tweeting their support using the hashtag #EqualPay.

In addition to the pay disparity, the USWNT has also faced discrimination in terms of working conditions and resources.

The team has had to fight for access to the same training facilities, travel, accommodation and medical resources as the men. The team's lawsuit alleged that this discrimination was a violation of the Equal Pay Act, which abolished pay gaps based on gender, and the Civil Rights Act, which outlawed discrimination for the same reason, as well as for race, skin colour, religion or birthplace.

In March 2021, the team reached a settlement with the USSF, which included provisions for equal travel allowances, hotel stays and staffing support. However, the settlement did not address the issue of equal pay, and the team's fight for equality continues. The team's former captain, Megan Rapinoe, has been perhaps the most vocal advocate on the issue, using her platform to raise awareness and call for change. In a statement following the team's settlement, she stated, "Equal pay is about more than just salaries; it's about respect, dignity and the right to be treated fairly."[91]

The grassroots mobilization and awareness spearheaded by the USWNT through social media showcases the tremendous positive impact it can have. However, the rise of social media also brings about complex new challenges. Regular users, particularly public figures such as elite athletes, confront threats to their mental wellbeing each time they log on to their social media accounts. Despite its importance, the #EqualPay movement encountered considerable and predictable backlash from online trolls. Yet, when utilized effectively, social media has the potential to revolutionize niche areas of the sporting world.

Traditionally, broadcasters have been conservative in their approach to choosing what they air, only offering content they believe will be successful, partly due to the high stakes involved. The democratization of media in general has transformed this landscape, allowing previously overlooked programming to flourish, find its audience and break into the mainstream.

However, this incredible accessibility comes with inherent problems, burdening individual athletes with the weight of its repercussions. I firmly believe that social media companies should bear the responsibility to protect end users from harmful content and hateful comments. But also, there is a degree of responsibility for us as users. We should not passively accept online hate as an inevitable reality and by-product of global connectivity. We must be willing to take action, even if it means abandoning platforms that fail to adhere to the standards we expect from them.

YOU CAN'T BE WHAT YOU CAN'T SEE

In addition to increased visibility, another factor driving the popularity of female sports is the rise of participation. In recent years, more women and girls have been encouraged to take part through groundbreaking campaigns, such as *This Girl Can*, which was launched in the UK in 2015 to negate athletic body-image standards and encourage everyone to play sports. Increased participation will help to create a larger pool of talented female athletes, leading to greater competitiveness and rising standards.

The increased popularity of women's sports has also led to greater investment and financial support. Major companies and brands are increasingly recognizing the potential of female athletes as marketing assets, leading to better sponsorship deals and endorsement opportunities. For example, Serena Williams, one of the greatest tennis players of all time, has signed lucrative deals with brands such as Nike, Gatorade and Wilson. In 2019 alone, Williams made

$32 million just in endorsements.[92] This was in addition to prize money and other sources of income.

However, Serena was the only female on the list of the top 50 of the world's highest-paid athletes of 2022.[93] She also competes in a sport which has blazed a trail in terms of female representation for longer and more authentically than almost any other. This highlights that, despite the progress that has been made over recent decades, there are still significant differences between men's and women's sports. Women's sports continue to receive less funding, less promotion and less media coverage than men's.

This can make participating in sport difficult, stressful and hard to manage for women with existing life, family and work commitments. Take the example of Natasha Thomas, the record goal-scorer for Ipswich Town women, and one of nine professional players on their books. Despite her sporting achievements, she needs to work 30–40 hours a week as a personal trainer to supplement her income.[94] Dividing her focus and energy is surely not helping her reach her sporting potential. It is also a world away from the experiences of a comparable male footballer.

The gender pay gap across sports can have various mental wellbeing consequences. Earning less money than male counterparts, despite achieving similar or even greater success, will naturally lead to feelings of undervaluation and diminished self-worth. It can understandably make female athletes question their skills, abilities and overall contribution to their sport.

Lower earnings naturally create financial burdens, making it harder for female athletes to meet their basic needs and pursue their athletic careers. This financial strain can also be a source of stress and anxiety, and create a sense of insecurity about an athlete's future. This ultimately creates a situation where many talented athletes can be put off pursuing a career in sport altogether.

Disparities in pay also inherently perpetuate the perception that women's sports are less important or of less worth. It's not hard to see how this can affect female athletes' sense of recognition and visibility, potentially leading to feelings of frustration, marginalization and decreased motivation. So, the gender pay gap in sports isn't solely an economic issue – it significantly affects mental wellbeing.

THE BEAUTY–PERFORMANCE PARADOX – WOMEN'S STRUGGLES IN SPORTS

One of the most significant pressures faced by female elite athletes is to conform to gender and beauty norms. In general, women are expected to be feminine, soft-spoken and nurturing, whereas athletes are expected to be strong, aggressive and competitive. These conflicting expectations can create stress and anxiety for female athletes, who may feel that they are not living up to societal expectations.

For example, female gymnasts are expected to be petite, flexible and graceful. But they also have to be strong and powerful enough to perform complex manoeuvres that push them to the very limit of what is possible from the human body. These competing narratives can lead to a range of issues, including body image concerns, eating disorders and other mental health struggles. It's not just gymnasts who face these types of problems. A study of female college athletes in the US found that 25 per cent of them reported disordered eating behaviours.[95]

We have established that social media has become an integral part of modern sporting culture. However, conversely, it can also be a source of immense pressure for female athletes. As Tayla Harris can attest, women are often judged on their appearance and perceived femininity, and social media can amplify these pressures.

On top of that, women are frequently judged more harshly than men and are held to a different standard of behaviour, just because of the gender norms that viewers project onto them. For example, female athletes may be criticized for being too aggressive or not feminine enough, while male athletes are praised for their toughness and competitiveness.

This double standard can have a significant impact on female athletes' mental health, as they may feel that they can never fully live up to the expectations placed on them. Serena Williams, one of the greatest tennis players of all time, faced criticism throughout her career for her aggressive style of play. Williams has spoken openly about the impact that these comments had on her mental health, admitting that she struggled with self-doubt and anxiety as a result.[96]

It's clear that female athletes face more than just performance pressure. Unrealistic expectations about their looks, behaviour, and femininity, often amplified by social media, play a big role in their mental health struggles. To create a healthier environment in sports, we need to challenge these double standards and offer better support systems that cater to both the physical and mental well-being of female athletes.

REPRESENTATION BEYOND THE FIELD

The struggle for female representation in sports extends beyond the field of play. Despite comprising nearly half of all football fans, women have long been underrepresented in sport media. A report by Women in Football revealed that only 12 per cent of sports journalists in the UK are women.[97] This lack of representation carries tangible consequences, as it subtly perpetuates the misconception that women's opinions on sports hold less significance than men's. As discussed, when it comes to the mental health revolution, women are equally as important, if not more so, in terms of driving the movement forward, so their voices are needed now more than ever.

When women do appear on screen, it can give the impression of tokenism. In reality, the women who do succeed in sports broadcasting usually have to far surpass standards set by their male counterparts. They do so knowing that their performance is under a microscope. Everything they say will be analysed and scrutinized. Any mistakes will be pounced upon. As Dr Grange asserts, "Across elite sport, I've spoken to a lot of very capable women who've told me how hard it is not to get pulled down by others' low expectations of what's possible in a male-dominated world. They know they are equal in intelligence, skill and character, but they also know that people often don't expect them to lead, raise their voices or take risks like their male counterparts."[98]

Football in the UK has been particularly slow to embrace gender diversity in the media. The industry has long been dominated by men. Women who do make it often face discrimination and harassment, with many facing gender-based abuse and sexism on a regular basis.

But in recent years, there has been a growing movement to change the status quo. As discussed already, women's football has seen a surge in popularity in the UK, with record-breaking attendances at matches and increased media coverage. This boost in interest has brought with it new opportunities for women to break into sports media and make their voices heard.

One key example of this change is The Women's Football Show, a weekly program dedicated to women's football on the BBC. The show features analysis and highlights from the Women's Super League, as well as interviews with players and coaches. The program has been widely praised for its in-depth coverage of women's football and its commitment to gender diversity in the media. A show dedicated to women's domestic football receiving mainstream coverage on the BBC was pretty much unthinkable a generation ago. Yet, it is visibility like this that is so crucial to driving genuine change.

There has also been a rise in female sports journalists and commentators. In the UK, women like Jacqui Oatley, Clare Balding and Gabby Logan have broken down barriers and paved the way for the next generation of women in the industry. These women are not only talented and knowledgeable, but they also serve as role models for young girls who aspire to work in sports media.

Still, there is work to be done. Among those few women that do make it into mainstream sports media, the treatment they are given is incomparable to their male counterparts. A prime example of this is the heated exchange on social media between former England footballer Karen Carney and Leeds United FC, which sparked a wave of controversy and criticism.

The incident began on 29 December 2020, when Carney, who is now a pundit for the BBC, made comments during a broadcast about Leeds United's promotion to the Premier League. Carney suggested that the Covid-19 pandemic and the subsequent break in the football season may have played a role in the team's success. She said, "They got promoted because of Covid... it gave them a bit of respite. I don't know if they'd have got up if they didn't have that break."[99]

The comments immediately drew backlash, with the Leeds United's official Twitter account issuing a response that was widely perceived as aggressive and confrontational. The tweet suggested that Carney had undermined the team's achievements, and pointed out they had, in fact, won the league by 10 points. Naturally, in the tribal and toxic atmosphere that surrounds football on social media, this induced a pile-on.

The situation quickly escalated, with Carney receiving a barrage of abusive and threatening messages. She eventually deleted her Twitter account, after revealing the extent of the personal abuse that she had received.

Carney's experience is yet another incident that highlights the broader issues around the treatment of women in sports media. Women in the industry have long faced discrimination, sexism and blocked pathways, and incidents like this only serve to reinforce the notion that women are not valued for their contributions in male-dominated spaces.

The fact that Carney was subjected to abuse and threats for simply doing her job is another reminder of the work that still needs to be done to create a more inclusive and equitable industry. I find it impossible to believe that any male pundit would have received the same amount of abuse that Carney suffered for expressing similar opinions. In fact, I know they wouldn't, because as much as I respect Carney as a pundit, the point she was making was not original. Many other commentators and former players had already made the very same point, that Leeds United's then-manager Marcelo Bielsa's style of hyper-intense training and pressing meant his players benefited from the mid-season Covid-enforced break. This perspective had been widely discussed before Carney mentioned it. However, none of those male pundits received anywhere near the same degree of abuse.

In the aftermath of the incident, there were calls for greater accountability from football clubs and governing bodies in the industry. Some argued that Leeds United's response was inappropriate, and that the club should have taken a more conciliatory approach, while others pointed to the wider culture of online abuse and harassment that needs to be addressed.

We are witnessing numerous incidents that highlight the dual nature of social media platforms. While they can serve as powerful tools for connecting fans and driving forward social causes, they unfortunately also foster an environment of abuse and harassment, particularly toward women.

As sports – and society as a whole – shift increasingly to online platforms, it is crucial that we take immediate action to establish safer and more inclusive spaces for all individuals involved. Failing to do so will result in an unwelcoming atmosphere that discourages some fans and players from participating at all. This lack of diversity in voice and opinion will be harmful for the sporting landscape. It also has the potential to set back some of the important groundwork that has been laid in the mental health revolution.

7

INJURY

... And Its Impact on Athletes' Mental Health

As I previously outlined, participating in sports offers numerous benefits, from physical fitness to personal development and team camaraderie. However, it is important to acknowledge that sport also comes with inherent risks, including the potential for injuries.

Governing bodies must take proactive measures to mitigate risks and ensure the safety of participants. Naturally, injury rates vary significantly depending on the type of sport, the level of competition and the individual athlete's characteristics.

Certain sports will always carry a higher risk of injury due to their nature, such as rugby or American football, which involve big physical collisions. On the other hand, sports like swimming or track and field generally have lower injury rates, due to their lack of contact.

Injury rate can even vary by gender. For example, there is ongoing research into the spate of ACL injuries suffered among female professional footballers. It is considered one of the worst injuries a footballer can suffer, and current data suggests that female players are 2.5 to 3.5 times more likely to suffer from it than their male counterparts.[100] However, due to the significant differences in resources between the men's and women's game, as covered in the last chapter, research on the issue is not as well developed or funded as one would hope.

While the physical effects of injuries are widely recognized and discussed, the psychological toll they take on athletes is often overlooked. Studies are emerging that explore the link between sports injuries and mental illness, finally emphasizing the need to address athletes' mental health alongside their physical wellbeing.

These studies consistently show that sports injuries are a significant risk factor for psychological distress and an increased risk of mental ill-health among athletes. Those who have experienced major negative life events, including severe injuries, are more likely to suffer from mental health issues, particularly depression.[101]

In a groundbreaking study exploring the link between mental health and injury in sportspeople, Amelia Gulliver from the Australian National University conclusively established a connection. Her research revealed that former athletes who had experienced severe injuries or undergone surgeries were up to seven times more likely to exhibit symptoms of common mental disorders, compared to those without injury or surgery. These results clearly prove the association between sports-related injuries and mental health issues within the athletic population.[102]

The emotional strain of dealing with an injury, combined with the physical limitations it imposes, can naturally contribute to feelings of sadness, anger and frustration. This perhaps comes as no surprise. As previously acknowledged, athletes dedicate their lives to their sports in order to reach the peak of their professions. Their performance is frequently a source of praise and adoration, which no doubt helps to reinforce their life decisions. However, injury strips away a fundamental aspect of athletes' identity and their system of rewards.

Too often, injuries are accepted as an inevitable part of sport, with a focus on the physical rather than the mental health considerations. Even healthcare professionals tend to concentrate solely on an athlete's physical training and competition demands, without paying enough attention to their mental wellbeing. But if we consider the mental strain athletes face and how it can affect injuries, we can create support systems during recovery to help ease their psychological burden. If we're going to accept injuries as part of the game, we should also do our best to lessen their mental toll.

For those who participate in a team sport, it is natural that injured players will feel a sense of separation from their teammates during recovery. Thankfully, clubs have become significantly better at keeping injured players engaged with the rest of the team than they were a few decades ago. There's proof of this in the example of Brian Clough, who served as a Nottingham Forest FC's manager from 1975 until 1993. Despite his reputation as one of the greatest managers of all time, he disregarded injured players. He deemed them as worthless and made them recover away from their teammates, as he didn't want them to impact the morale of the fit players he had at his disposal.[103] This neglectful attitude almost certainly further exacerbated the psychological struggles of those recovering from injuries.

Today, thankfully, most clubs are eager to offer injured players companionship and support. Understanding the emotional and psychological impact of being sidelined, clubs now prioritize the provision of a supportive environment to help injured players feel connected and included. By fostering a sense of togetherness, clubs aim to mitigate feelings of isolation, and ensure that injured players remain an integral part of the team, both on and off the field.

But what about those that compete as athletes in individual sports? Remember, as Frank Bruno said, "Boxing is the toughest and loneliest sport in the world" – that is doubly so for those who are injured. Recovery is psychologically challenging enough for athletes. Without a support network, it can become insurmountable and, in some instances, completely derail a career.

Though we have made some progress in the level of psychological support for injured athletes, it seems that there is further scope to improve provisions. The care of injured players should include skilled mental health professionals or specialized multidisciplinary teams, working alongside physiotherapists who support with physical recovery. Collaboration with psychologists or mental health practitioners can provide comprehensive support, enabling the identification of mental health concerns among injured athletes, and ultimately lead to a more holistic recovery.

Integrating both physical and mental components into rehabilitation proves to be the most effective method in facilitating athletes' physical recovery. This multidisciplinary approach is increasingly becoming the norm within sports, particularly within teams that possess substantial financial resources; in a sense they have finally grasped the significance of prioritizing the wellbeing of their key assets. However, as previously mentioned, it raises the question of how we can safeguard athletes participating in individual sports or those competing in sports with limited financial resources.

COPING WITH INJURY AND MENTAL HEALTH IN SPORTS

Mark Cavendish, a renowned British professional road-racing cyclist, is celebrated for his extraordinary sprinting prowess and remarkable success in prestigious cycling events. Cavendish has claimed numerous world championship titles, but his exploits in the Tour de France, the most iconic bike race of all, set him apart.

Participating as a sprinter in Grand Tour cycling events is one of the most curious undertakings in professional sport. Sprinters primarily target shorter, flatter stages conducive to electric finishes, as these athletes specialize in explosive bursts of speed. However, in the meantime, they still need to complete the long and mountainous stages within the qualification time to remain in the race, stretches that are completely unsuited to their sprinting skill set. In other words, it's like asking Usain Bolt to run a marathon nearly every day for a month, interspersed with sporadic 100-meter races.

Between 2008 and 2016, Cavendish won a remarkable 30 individual Tour stages, which made him the second-most successful athlete in terms of individual stage wins, just behind the legendary Belgian cyclist Eddy Merckx, who won 34. As Cavendish was only 30 and at the top of his profession, it seemed almost inevitable that Merckx's benchmark, which had stood for more than 40 years, would be toppled.

By 2017, needing just four stage wins to equal Merckx's record, Cavendish was once again among the favourites to bring home more victories. However, during stage four of the Tour, a moment occurred that would forever change the trajectory of his career. As the frontrunners fiercely sprinted toward the finish line, Cavendish became entangled in a chaotic jostle for position. In a moment of intense competition, he was struck by a forceful elbow from rival Peter Sagan. The impact sent Cavendish hurtling toward the crash barrier at a staggering speed of about 40mph. The ensuing chaos saw a pack of racers unable to evade him, riding directly over Cavendish's head in the aftermath of the collision. Afterwards, Cavendish was forced out of the Tour with a broken shoulder, and Sagan was also disqualified for endangering a fellow rider.

Less than a year later, Cavendish rode in the classic race, Milan–San Remo. His return was marred by yet another dramatic crash. Cavendish flipped headfirst over his handlebars after crashing into a traffic bollard. Some critics argued that his comeback was premature, questioning whether he had fully recovered. Others speculated that his once-sharp reflexes and skills had permanently declined. Either way, Cavendish struggled to regain his form, and he found himself grappling with strained relationships, both within his team and with his family, which neared breaking point.

One thing I really admire about Mark Cavendish is how, despite living in a time when athletes are trained from a young age to handle the media, he stays refreshingly unpolished. He's had his share of clashes with the press. Once, a journalist asked if he was "100 per cent sure that no riders in the sport were on drugs". In reply, a frustrated Cavendish said, "Can you tell me 100 per cent that one of these journalists isn't fucking your wife?"[104]

Following the crash in the Milan–San Remo, on the 2018 Tour de France, Cavendish was timed out, missing the cut on a mountainous stage 11, coming in around an hour behind the leading pack. As his form dipped, patience wore thin, particularly with his general manager at Team Dimension Data, Doug Ryder, who dropped Cavendish altogether for the 2019 Tour. The relationship between Ryder and Cavendish had been challenging at the best of times. Now that Cavendish was out of form and perceived as on the decline, Ryder wasted little time in shutting him out of the most illustrious event on the cycling calendar. It appears that when you're at the top of your profession and your career is filled with successes, you're given much more leeway for being confrontational compared to when you're not achieving the same level of success.

During this period, Cavendish was also diagnosed with Epstein-Barr virus, a condition known for inducing chronic fatigue. This diagnosis essentially made it impossible for him to compete at the highest level of the sport.

When you distil the essence of what defines great athletes, their need to win often lies at the heart of their character. When you strip that away, what is left? In the case of Mark Cavendish, his identity was winning bike races. Through a combination of injury and viral infection, he was rapidly having to learn what life was like when that was no longer the case.

To cope with his diminishing performance, Cavendish began restricting his food intake. Initially aiming to achieve a lighter weight to enhance his speed, this endeavour soon escalated into a severe eating disorder, as he sought a degree of control over a life and career that was rapidly going off the rails.

By his own admission, Cavendish was not a fan of sports psychologists. They made him nervous. After all, he had largely succeeded throughout his career without relying on them. However, as injuries took their toll and his struggles with disordered eating intensified, he finally sought help.

He received a diagnosis of depression, which posed a fundamental challenge to the core principles of his identity. He had always viewed himself as immune to such struggles, believing it was something that afflicted others. For him, depression was the kind of thing that affected individuals who lacked the resilience and determination that had defined his character and propelled him to success. And yet, he found himself facing it head-on, confronting a reality he never imagined he would encounter.

Injury can fundamentally rob athletes of a perspective of who they are. As Cavendish himself said, "You don't go from being the best in the world, to nothing."[105] The abrupt transition can be overwhelming, even for those perceived as physically and mentally resilient. In Cavendish's case, by 2021, four years after his first career-changing crash, he found himself as the third-choice sprinter on the Quick-Step team, seemingly relegated to competing in minor tours as his career appeared to be on the wind-down. However, a surprising turn of events occurred when an unexpected injury opened a spot for him in the 2021 Tour de France.

Despite not initially being slated to compete, Cavendish had been quietly preparing behind the scenes as if he were going to take part. This preparation paid off handsomely. Against the odds, he clinched a stunning victory in stage 4 of the race, a triumph that felt almost like a fairy tale. Despite being written off by many, and after battling through so many adversities, Cavendish had once again won a stage on the tour, five years since his last.

The story didn't end there. Cavendish went on to win stages 6 and 10 as well, catapulting him from the depths of uncertainty to within striking distance of Eddy Merckx's Tour record. At stage 13, he duly equalled the Belgian, cementing the comeback as one of the most remarkable and inspiring narratives on the history of the tour.

He narrowly missed out taking the lead in overall stage wins during the final race of the 2021 Tour, the iconic finale along the Champs-Élysées in Paris. Cavendish then joined the Astana team. However, after being not being selected to ride the Tour in 2022, and not taking a stage win in 2023, it seemed that he would forever be tied with Merckx. Perhaps there was something poetic about sharing the record. After all, having gone through everything that Cavendish had, there was some comfort in knowing that he was not on his own.

However, 16 years after his first, and eight hard years since his 30th stage win, Cavendish finally took the record 35th stage victory. He is immortalized in the race's history as its greatest-ever stage winner. Thankfully, the post-race comments also suggest a much more content and grounded individual than earlier in his career. Enjoying the moment, he reflected, "What's the point in doing anything unless you can share it with those people close to you?"[106] Having, battled through illness, crashes and non-selection, Mark Cavendish stands alone as the all-time Tour de France stage-win record holder. No doubt the dark times that he struggled through made his historic achievement all the sweeter.

THE LINK BETWEEN SPORTING-INDUCED BRAIN INJURY AND MENTAL HEALTH

The risk of head injuries in sport, particularly concussions, has become a subject of fierce debate. In recent years, the inherent safety of contact sports like American football and rugby has been questioned, even bringing the future viability of those sports into question.

Recent findings from the Boston University CTE Center have brought to light the concerning connection between American football and Chronic Traumatic Encephalopathy (CTE).[107] CTE is a progressive and fatal brain disease associated with repeated traumatic brain injuries, including concussions and repeated blows to the head. The disease is characterized by the presence of misfolded tau protein, distinct from changes associated with ageing, Alzheimer's disease or other brain disorders. However, it *is* associated with the development of dementia.[108]

Their study revealed that out of 376 former National Football League (NFL) players studied, an astonishing 345 players (91.7 per cent), were diagnosed with CTE. This includes well-known figures like Rick Arrington, who was a quarterback for the Philadelphia Eagles, and Ed Lothamer, a defensive tackle for the Kansas City Chiefs.[109]

To put these figures into perspective, a comparable study examining 164 brains among members of the public, found that only 0.6 per cent (1 out of 164) had traces of CTE. This single case was that of a former college football player. These numbers align with similar studies conducted by brain banks in Austria, Australia and Brazil, all finding a low prevalence of CTE within the general population.[110]

The research is increasingly clear: repetitive head impacts are the primary risk factor for CTE. To gain a deeper understanding of CTE and develop effective diagnostic and treatment methods, Dr Ann McKee, director of the Boston University CTE Center, is actively inviting former athletes to participate in research studies at the time of writing this book.

Former Philadelphia Eagles quarterback and ESPN sideline reporter Rick Arrington suffered from the effects of CTE for 35 years before his death in 2021. His daughter Jill shared her personal experience and highlighted the importance of contributing to the research that McKee and others are doing. She believes her father's true legacy lies in his decision to donate his brain, and she urges all former football players to consider participating in the study.

One of the most well-known cases of CTE involves Aaron Hernandez. Hernandez showed exceptional athletic talent from a young age, particularly in American football. He played in college for the Florida Gators and helped secure the team's victory in the BCS National Championship in 2008. Although he caught the eye of many NFL franchises during his college years, his time at the University of Florida was also marred by off-field troubles. He was embroiled in scandals related to drugs and violence. These lingering problems meant some teams avoided him during the 2010 NFL Draft, despite his obvious talent. But the New England Patriots decided to take a chance on him, selecting him in the fourth round.

He wasted no time leaving his mark on the field, showcasing his versatility and earning recognition for his athleticism and skilful play. Alongside fellow tight end Rob Gronkowski, Hernandez became part of a formidable duo in the Patriots' offense, contributing to the team's journey to Super Bowl XLVI in 2012. He even snagged a touchdown pass from Tom Brady in the big game, although his team would eventually lose to the New York Giants.

He seemed to be destined for a long and successful career in the NFL. However, off the field, Hernandez's image continued to be tarnished by the same types of controversies that dogged his college years. This culminated in 2013, when he was arrested and charged with the murder of his friend Odin Lloyd, a semi-professional American football player. Despite maintaining his innocence, Hernandez was found guilty of first-degree murder in 2015 and sentenced to life in prison without the possibility of parole. Just two years into his sentence, Hernandez died by suicide, at the age of just 27. His brain was then donated to the Boston University CTE Centre.[111]

In 2017, Dr McKee and her team revealed shocking findings from their examination of Hernandez's brain: he had the most severe case of CTE ever observed in someone of his age. He was suffering from Stage 3 CTE, which researchers had never seen in someone who was under 46 years old. The experts at Boston University emphasized that the extent of brain damage would have profoundly impacted his ability to make decisions, exercise judgement and process information.[112]

From an external perspective, Hernandez's brain appeared unremarkable. It didn't have any visible bruises or irregularities. However, when the team at Boston University sliced the brain into sections and studied it more closely, they made a series of alarming discoveries that perhaps hint at the root cause of Hernandez's erratic behaviour. The ventricles in his brain had expanded, a sign that his brain had shrunk. Structural components that should have been robust exhibited a thin and jelly-like consistency, and notable holes were found throughout certain regions of the brain. Key areas vital for cognitive function showed significant deterioration, too. The hippocampus, crucial for memory processes, had diminished in size. The fornix, another contributor to memory, had undergone atrophy. Furthermore, the frontal lobe, essential for higher cognitive functions, such as problem-solving and social behaviour, exhibited tau protein deposits resembling pockmarks. Lastly, the amygdala, pivotal for emotional regulation and fear response, displayed severe impairment.[113]

Some will point to Hernandez's checkered past as evidence that he was just a troubled individual to whom something bad would inevitably happen. However, given the scale of scientific evidence coming out of the Boston University CTE Center's studies, it is increasingly hard to ignore the role that repeated concussive blows caused by playing American football had on his brain. The sport therefore must be at least partly responsible for the deaths of both Aaron Hernandez and Odin Lloyd.

Thanks to the ongoing work that Dr McKee and her team are conducting, our knowledge of CTE is constantly growing. However, as we strive for a potential cure for CTE, or at least a way of managing the very worst aspects of this disease, it also raises questions about the viability of sports that frequently induce concussions. Much of the data is from the NFL, but CTE is by no means limited to American football. Former England rugby player Steve Thompson recently disclosed that he is suffering from early onset dementia. Reflecting on his team's victory in the 2003 World Cup final, he revealed that he couldn't remember being at the game at all. Additionally, he admitted that he could not recall the scores from a single game in his career.[114] Thompson is not an old man – at the time of this interview, he was 42.

Around the same time, Ryan Jones, a former Wales rugby international and peer of Thompson, revealed that he too is suffering from early onset dementia, thought to be brought on by CTE. There are also numerous examples from other contact sports, including boxing, football, ice hockey, mixed martial arts and Australian rules football.

Insurmountable evidence is piling up that sports that lead to contact with the head and cause frequent concussions are triggers for severe mental health issues and brain diseases. How could this not be a challenge for the very existence of those sports?

As we saw in the case of Aaron Hernandez, the link between American football and CTE poses a significant risk, not only to the players themselves, but also to the people around them. Despite efforts by the NFL to mitigate head trauma, the very nature of American football makes concussions nearly unavoidable. Although the league has introduced rule changes and protocols to address concussions, there remains a persistent risk.

The NFL, as a governing body, has been accused of prioritizing its own interests over player safety. In the past, the NFL has staunchly denied the connection between the sport and CTE. However, in 2015, as evidence began to mount, the league settled a class-action lawsuit brought by former players. Ultimately, they agreed to pay up to $1 billion in medical costs for 20,000 current and former players affected by concussions and potential CTE-related problems.

While American football provides thrilling entertainment, how can it justify the risks posed to players' lives and wellbeing?

The growing evidence of American football's harmful effects on players' health has led to a decline in youth participation in the sport, as parents become more hesitant to expose their children to these risks. A study in Arizona found that in just two years, there was a 17-point decrease in the percentage of parents willing to let their child play contact sports.[115] Naturally, parents are becoming increasingly wary of exposing their children to a sport directly linked with severe brain trauma. Based on pure logic, the future of contact-based sports like American football are uncertain at best and, at worst, completely unviable. Yet, sport very rarely occupies the territory of pure logic.

It appears quite likely that sports like American football will never be banned, at least not in my lifetime. Although it doesn't have the worldwide appeal of football (soccer), NFL franchises are incredibly powerful money-making entities. In fact, the top three most valuable sports franchises in the world are all NFL teams.[116]

Also, like many other athletes, American footballers are extremely well paid. The average salary in the NFL is $2.7 million per year.[117] At the time of writing this book, the highest paid player in the league, quarterback Joe Burrow, is paid $62.9 million per year by the Cincinnati Bengals.[118] With the potential glory, sporting immortality and riches on offer, there will probably always be a carousel of young men who are willing to put their bodies and brains on the line for an NFL contract.

With all this said, it is evident that there is at least a greater need in high-contact sports to prioritize the wellbeing of athletes. Stricter safety measures, enhanced protective equipment and improved training techniques are just a few areas that require attention.

It is crucial that those in charge of sport governing bodies, like the NFL, no longer bury their heads in the sand. Rather than waiting for insurmountable evidence before acting, it should be in their interests to mitigate the long-term consequences of head impacts and ensure a safer future for athletes of all ages and genders. Otherwise, the existential threat to contact sports could come home to roost.

Finally, subjecting high-profile athletes to CTE-inducing brain injuries increases the likelihood of them experiencing extreme and sudden changes in behaviour, potentially leading to violent acts, such as those perpetrated by Aaron Hernandez. This issue also poses a challenge in the context of the ongoing mental health revolution. When irreversible brain damage is not fully understood, it can unfairly cast the sufferer in a barbaric light. In the case of Aaron Hernandez, his actions on the surface are utterly unforgivable. However, as we delve deeper into the complexities of CTE, the moral judgement becomes increasingly complex.

As much as I cherish the world of sports, I find it increasingly difficult to reconcile the idea of exposing players to irreversible brain damage while simultaneously advocating for a mental health revolution.

8

THE HIDDEN OPPONENT

The Very Darkest Side of Sport

WHEN THE GAME ENDS – ATHLETES, SUICIDE AND MENTAL HEALTH

Suicide is a complex phenomenon with multiple causes, and it is often the result of a combination of factors. While mental illness is one of the leading causes of suicide, it is by no means the only reason. People who suffer from these conditions can be more susceptible to experiencing feelings of hopelessness and despair, which can lead to suicidal thoughts and behaviours.

When famous athletes take their own lives, it is incredibly shocking. We tend to think of these sports stars as superhuman, untouched by the problems regular folks deal with. Sportspeople are often loved by many and earn enormous salaries. But the truth is, mental health issues and other factors that lead to suicide can hit anyone. Sadly, there have been quite a few tragic instances where sports stars have died by suicide. This includes well-known figures like footballers Robert Enke and Gary Speed, and ice hockey players Wade Belak and Tom Cavanagh, among others.

Some, like Enke, opened up about their struggles with depression to their loved ones, but also lived in fear of the repercussions of it becoming public knowledge. Enke's father, Dirk, admitted in the aftermath of his son's death that "during the most critical phases, Robert would have a fear of the ball coming near his goal. He had attacks, he didn't want to go to training... He was always very close to taking this step, to be admitted to hospital."[119] However, Enke also worried about what impact being sectioned would have on his career. He thought it would essentially mean the end of professional football for him – the one thing he loved and was good at.

On the other hand, in the case of legendary Welsh footballer Gary Speed, his choice to end his life seemingly came with little warning. In the months leading up to his death, Speed had been prescribed antidepressants and was reportedly seeking therapy. However, he gave no outward signs of his inner turmoil, and his death came as a shock to his friends, family and fans.

THE LOST TALENT – JEREMY WISTEN'S STORY

Speed and Enke were both players who had scaled the very heights of professional football, representing their countries and some of the biggest clubs in the world. However, on 24 October 2020, the football world was rocked by the news of the death of a player most fans had never heard of. Jeremy Wisten was an 18-year-old former Manchester City Academy player who died by suicide after struggling with mental health issues following his release from the club.

Born in Malawi, Wisten moved to the UK with his family at a young age and quickly developed a passion for football. He joined the Manchester City Academy at the age of 13 and established himself as a talented young player. However, his dreams of a career in football were shattered when he suffered a serious injury that kept him out of action for several months.

Despite his best efforts to return to the field, Wisten was released by the club in 2020, leaving him devastated and struggling with his mental health, eventually leading to his death.

His family released a statement in which they expressed their grief and called for increased mental health support for young footballers, as Wisten told them that he felt he hadn't received sufficient support from his former club. They accused Manchester City of not doing enough to support him in finding a new club, and opined that the club could have done more – and that they had indeed done more for others.[120]

Wisten's death is now part of a wider conversation about the mental health challenges faced by young footballers, and the need for clubs to provide adequate support, particularly among those that don't make it – and the vast majority do not make it.

In England, for example, the Premier League has conducted research that shows that less than 1 per cent of players who join a Premier League academy at the age of 9 or 10 will go on to become professional footballers. This statistic applies to all clubs in the Premier League, and the numbers are even lower for professional academies at lower levels of the footballing pyramid.

The Premier League's research also revealed that only around 180 of the 1.5 million boys who play organized youth football in England every year will sign professional contracts with Premier League clubs.[121] This means that the chances of a young player making it to the very top of the game are extremely slim – 0.0001 per cent, to be precise.

So, what happens to those who *don't* make it – and are clubs doing enough to adequately prepare them for life and alternative careers?

In response to Wisten's death, Manchester City released a statement expressing their condolences, stating that they were committed to providing support to their players.[122] Yet, many people find it hard to swallow that Manchester City, a club known for spending tens, if not hundreds of millions of pounds on transfers every year, are not doing a better job looking after their young academy players. It's only fair to expect better support for those who don't make the cut, especially from a rich club like Manchester City. However, the challenge of providing that care is huge, if we think about the massive number of kids who go through professional sports academies, versus the tiny fraction who actually make it as professionals.

Sarah Nightingale, who takes care of player support at Cardiff City Football Club, admits that looking after everyone is challenging. She says, "It's about being smart with the system. The big changes happen for the under-18s and under-21s, especially when we have to let them go. That's when they really need our help and support. It's tougher with the under 15s. We do keep in touch with those whose parents want us to, we try and support them with finding new clubs. However, quite a few parents turn around and say, 'We don't want your support.'"[123]

With the sheer number of boys and girls that come through the doors of professional clubs, it is a challenge to identify any red flags or potential issues. That is why people like Nightingale are increasingly questioning the pre-existing cultures and methods deployed in academies. She is challenging academy managers and the coaching staff to change the culture within youth sport. She says they can do this "by questioning if they are just selecting someone to make up the numbers of the scholarships, or if they genuinely believe they have a future in football. Because, if the answer is no, then why are we putting them through this?"[124] This fresh approach and honesty doesn't always make her popular with more traditional coaches, yet it also hints at the increasing number of people within professional sports who are putting the mental health of participants ahead of the system.

I know there are a lot of very good people who look out for the interests of young players within the developmental pathways of sporting institutions. Yet, critics will argue that more needs to be done to support them, particularly in the light of incidents such as the case of Jeremy Wisten. What is clear is that clubs and governing bodies need to provide more than just lip service when it comes to mental health support. We need to see a culture shift in football, with clubs investing in mental health support and creating a safe environment for players of all ages.

It is a tragedy that Wisten had to die to bring to light the mental health challenges faced by young footballers. This situation also shows that clubs have a duty to look after everyone in their system, not just those who make it to the professional ranks. If clubs keep tempting countless young players with dreams of fame, knowing most won't succeed, they must help support those who don't make it. They should put the mental health and wellbeing of these young athletes first. The biggest clubs and governing bodies surely have the means to offer more support in this area.

There's a well-known quote from Bill Shankly, the iconic former Liverpool FC manager, who said, "Football isn't a matter of life and death, it's more important than that."[125]

However, I am sure that in the face of these tragedies, Shankly would revise his opinion. Instead, I tend to think along the lines of legendary Italian manager, Arrigo Sacchi that football is "the most important of the unimportant things in life."[126] This is a much healthier way of understanding football and sports in general. I am certain that many players and fans alike could enjoy several mental health benefits by keeping things in this perspective.

The tragic cases of Jeremy Wisten, along with Robert Enke and Gary Speed, underscore the critical need for a mental health revolution in sports. These athletes' struggles highlight the importance of creating an open dialogue about mental health, led by athletes themselves. We need to create a supportive space where people can openly share what they're going through without feeling alone. Knowing that others understand and have been through the same can be a huge help and might even save lives. This push for change is all about making sure athletes at every level get the support and help they need to take care of their mental health, so, if possible, we can avoid such heartbreaking events in the future.

UNRAVELLING THE TRAGEDY – THE CHRIS BENOIT STORY

I'm not going to dedicate too much time to whether professional wrestling is a sport or not. For the sake of this book, I'm just going to come down on the side of the fence that it is.

Like many people my age who were fortunate enough to have parents who were early adopters of cable television, I was pretty much obsessed with the World Wrestling Federation

(WWF), now called World Wrestling Entertainment (WWE). When I watched, it was the golden era of wrestling. A cast of obscenely colourful characters like Hulk Hogan, "Macho Man" Randy Savage and The Ultimate Warrior competed in the sport, grappling in exaggerated choreographed combat in little more than florescent underpants.

I eventually drifted away from it in my early teens, when it started to feel a little embarrassing for me to watch the sport and all of its predetermined outcomes. (This isn't a judgement on any adult wrestling fans, of course.) Even with the choreographed fights and mapped-out storylines, it is undeniable that wrestlers possess impressive physical prowess, and require immense dedication to reach the pinnacle of the sport. However, wrestling, perhaps more than any other sport, has been marred by tragic cases. This may be attributed to its unique nature. I believe its status as a quasi-sport opens it up to several factors that become a potent cocktail of mental health issues.

Wrestling is first and foremost an entertainment product mixed with combat sport, which naturally leads to physically imposing and muscular competitors being preferable. Also, with the results being predetermined, there is not the degree of true competition you see in other sports. In the '80s and '90s in particular, this led to a casual acceptance of steroid use.

The biggest star of this era of wrestling was Hulk Hogan, an industry legend who has been in the public eye since the 1970s. He is widely regarded as one of the most influential wrestlers of all time and has been a household name for decades. Hogan is known for his impressive size and strength, charismatic personality and larger-than-life persona, mixing his powerful, high impact moves with a dose of all-American jingoism. Watching his performances back, his true skill was his ability to connect with the crowd, often whipping them into a frenzy with his signature catchphrases and posing routines.

To put it mildly, Hogan was a physical specimen. His biceps were absolutely enormous. This was achieved not just through exercise and diet, but also through the habitual use of anabolic steroids. Hogan later admitted that steroids were an integral part of the game. He said, "In the '70s and '80s, doctors would write you a prescription for a steroid; every sport in the world was doing it. The mindset was, it was safer than taking sugar... I would tell kids to train, say their prayers and take their vitamins. But it wasn't just vitamins I was taking."[127]

This also brings us to the toll that wrestling puts on competitors' bodies. While professional wrestling is scripted and the outcomes are pre-planned, the physical demands and risks associated with the sport are real.

Wrestlers put themselves through intense training and perform physically demanding moves that can result in injuries. Furthermore, unlike other combat sports where competitors will typically compete only a handful of times each year, wrestlers will perform week in and week out. This is particularly problematic when it comes to head injuries and concussions. It is not uncommon for wrestlers to suffer concussions and other types of brain injuries as a result of the sport's physical nature. For example, one common move in professional wrestling involves hitting an opponent in the head with a steel chair conveniently placed next to the ring. While this move is often staged and not intended to cause real harm, it can still result in serious head injuries.

It is this blend of drugs, head injuries and the toll of an unforgiving schedule that leads to professional wrestling being so dangerous for its performers. There are several online articles and fan sites dedicated to dead wrestlers, with the most common causes of death being drug overdoses, heart attacks and death by suicide. It seems that not too many wrestlers make it to a ripe old age. And still, in a sport littered with tragedy, one case stands out above the rest: Chris Benoit.

Chris Benoit was a talented Canadian professional wrestler who competed in various top promotions, including the WWE, World Championship Wrestling (WCW) and New Japan Pro-Wrestling (NJPW). On 25 June 2007, Benoit killed his wife Nancy and their seven-year-old son, Daniel, before taking his own life in their home in Fayetteville, Georgia. The incident shocked the world of professional wrestling and led to intense scrutiny of the industry's culture, including the use of steroids and other performance-enhancing drugs, the toll of a rigorous travel schedule, and the mental and emotional strain of the sport.

Due to the horrific nature of his crimes, those associated with WWE today are reluctant to talk about Benoit. However, based purely on wrestling ability, he is widely regarded as one of the greatest to ever compete. Former professional wrestler and colleague of Benoit Dean Malenko noted that "the act of what he did is unthinkable, unforgivable. But it's still hard for me to separate a friendship that I had with him... I will always look at Chris as one of the best performers our business has ever seen, and I'll just leave it at that."[128]

The media initially blamed steroids for the tragedy after a toxicology report found that Benoit had ten times the normal amount of testosterone in his body when he died.[129] However, in hindsight, this appears to be just one part of the puzzle.

It was later discovered that Benoit had been suffering from CTE, the very same disease that affects so many NFL alumni, and it is believed that the damage to his brain likely contributed to his actions on that tragic day. Another former WWE superstar, Chris Nowinski, is now a neuroscientist and runs the Concussion Legacy Foundation. At the time of Benoit's death, he was adamant that the deceased wrestler's brain should be tested for CTE. Six months before his death, Benoit had actually told Nowinski that he had endured a multitude of concussions throughout his wrestling career, so many that he couldn't even count them all. This revelation draws alarming parallels to the consistent concussions suffered by NFL players – and the end of Benoit's story is reminiscent of others we've already discussed in this book, such as Aaron Hernandez.

Benoit suffered countless chair-shots to the head during his career. On top of that, one of his signature moves was the flying headbutt. This involved standing on the top rope of the ring, flying high through the air headfirst, and headbutting an opponent, who would be laid prone on the canvas. This is a move that Benoit would have performed thousands of times, night after night throughout his career. It's hard to believe that this move was not at least partly responsible for the brain damage that he suffered.

Nowinski contacted the Benoit family for permission to check his brain for CTE damage. It quickly became apparent that Benoit suffered from a severe case of CTE. Nowinski stated, "There was damage in areas that you would think could influence emotional behaviour. I believe the degradation to his brain changed who he was and what he was capable of. If you get hit in the head thousands of times, your brain can essentially start to rot."[130]

The incident led to changes in WWE's policies, including the banning of the chair-shot to the head and the institution of a comprehensive drug-testing program. It also prompted increased research and awareness of CTE and its effects on athletes in various sports.

I never met Chris Benoit, and there's no excusing what he did. But from what his closest friends say, his actions didn't match the person they knew. His long-time wrestling partner and friend Chris Jericho noted, "Chris was always very much a great father. Very much about his family."[131]

The tragic Benoit case seems to demonstrate that mental health is not a constant, fixed point, but rather a dynamic and ever-changing state that requires ongoing care and nourishment. Just like our physical health, our mental health can be influenced by various factors, such as life events, stress, injury and trauma. Wrestling may seem like light entertainment, but at one time, the mixture of performance-enhancing drugs and regular concussive blows to the head made it uniquely dangerous for competitors. I understand and appreciate the appeal of the sport, but competitors must not be expected to sacrifice so much of themselves for their profession. Thankfully, now that we have greater regulation in place, I am hopeful that it will prevent another case like Benoit's from ever happening again.

Chris Benoit, like NFL tight end Aaron Hernandez, suffered irreversible damage due to the nature of his sport. It made him a danger not only to himself, but also to those around him. When some sports stars are seen as dangerous or barbaric, they risk tarnishing the reputation of athletes overall. Their cases may give ammunition to those with an anti-sport agenda, who will then push back against sportspeople in the very important battle to destigmatize mental health issues, thus creating a hurdle in the athlete-led mental health revolution. To stop this from happening, we need to protect competitors from the dangerous side effects of competition, such as CTE, and prevent tragedies like these from ever taking place again. That way, athletes can maintain their physical health – and encourage others to improve their mental health, too.

9

RETIREMENT

The Only Inevitable for Any Athlete

Retirement from professional sports can have a profound impact on the mental health and overall wellbeing of former athletes. Recent findings from a survey conducted by the Professional Players' Federation (PPF) shed light on this issue, revealing that more than half of retired athletes have grappled with concerns regarding their mental and emotional health after bidding farewell to their sporting careers.[132] Strikingly, this statistic closely aligns with the number of athletes within the Canadian Olympic program who received mental health-related diagnoses while still active in their respective sports.

Many athletes use the extreme dedication and focus needed for top-level sports to push aside their mental health issues. Unfortunately, these suppressed feelings can come to the surface when the structure of professional sports is then removed from their lives. Likewise, a lot of athletes talk about feeling lost, regretful and heartbroken as they try to navigate their lives post-retirement.

The PPF survey, which included responses from 800 former players across various sports, highlighted the significant psychological challenges faced by athletes after retirement.

Within two years of retiring, half admitted to feeling a lack of control over their lives.[133]

The transition from professional sports to a post-athletic life can be particularly daunting, as retirement often occurs in an athlete's thirties. This is the time in life where professionals in most other walks of life are getting a stronger foothold in their careers. For athletes, it's the exact opposite – a moment of great uncertainty and the daunting prospect of having to start again. Yes, we see many athletes go on to have highly visible careers in the media after their "first" career in sport. However, the chances of landing one of these roles are even smaller than the improbable odds of becoming a professional athlete in the first place, due to the incredibly small number of media jobs available.

Former athletes have spoken about the loss of identity they experience when they can no longer compete. Simon Taylor, the chief executive of the PPF, noted that it is not uncommon for athletes to express feelings of mourning and grief upon retiring.[134] The structure, purpose and validation that come with being a professional athlete suddenly disappear, leaving a void that can lead to profound psychological challenges. Retirement from sport can indeed have such an impact on an athlete that it can completely transform aspects of their lives, ones that are seemingly unrelated to their athletic pursuits.

Take the example of Jonathan Edwards. Edwards is a former triple jumper who won gold medals at the Olympics, World Championships and Commonwealth Games. At the time of writing, he is still the world record holder in his event for his jump of 18.29 metres (about 60 feet), a mark he set in 1995 that has not been beaten in nearly three decades.

While in the spotlight as a top-ranking triple jumper, Edwards was famously a Christian. Early in his career, his devotion was so strong that he refused to jump on Sundays. This meant he even missed out on the opportunity to medal at some of the most prestigious events in the athletics calendar.

Edwards's faith was also a central part of his athletic rituals. Prior to each competition, he began with the same prayer: "I place my destiny in your hands. Do with me as You will."[135] Considering the remarkable extent of success that Edwards achieved, it's reasonable to speculate that his faith was at least helpful in his athletic pursuits. After all, there is some research suggesting that individuals with strong faith are more likely to survive or recover from diseases.[136] If faith can have such a positive impact on overcoming a life-threatening illness, it stands to reason that it could also contribute to Jonathan Edwards gaining those extra centimetres in the triple jump – and I say that as a non-believer.

Due to his achievement in the triple jump, Edwards was widely regarded as one of the most well-known Christians in the UK. He continued his calling after retirement from athletics by taking on hosting duties of *Songs of Praise*, the most high-profile religious TV programme in the UK.

Yet, retirement from sport is transformative. Edwards himself admitted that he never doubted his belief in God for a single moment until he retired from sport. But when he retired, something happened that took him by complete surprise. He quickly realized that athletics were more important to his identity than he believed possible. He was the best in the world at what he did, and suddenly that was not true anymore. With one facet of his identity stripped away, he began to question the others, and from there, there was no stopping. The foundations of his world were slowly crumbling. He eventually had to confess that he "no longer believed."[137]

On the surface, a cynic may suggest that Edwards used his belief as a shield against pressure during his athletic career, only to drop Christianity when it was no longer necessary. And yet, an investigation into the facts seems to unveil a genuine loss of faith. Firstly, as discussed, Edwards left several major competition medals on the table early in his career due to his decision not to compete on Sundays.

Furthermore, Edwards also had to sacrifice his post-athletic career as host of *Songs of Praise* after admitting he was no longer Christian. It also put considerable strain on his personal life, as he was married to someone who also shared his previous religious conviction. I think it is clear that Edwards had a deep and strong faith throughout his career. Yet, the aftershocks of retirement had such a great impact that it led to a profound change in one of the cornerstones of his life.

The struggles faced by retired athletes extend beyond a loss of identity. The PPF survey revealed that many former players encounter serious mental health issues, such as depression, self-harm, addiction and financial problems. The single-minded pursuit of success during their sporting careers often leaves little room for planning and preparing for life after retirement, further complicating the transition process.

In recent years, sport governing bodies have increasingly acknowledged the importance of offering enhanced support to athletes as they transition into post-sport life. The Duty of Care In Sport Review by Baroness Grey-Thompson, part of the UK Government's sports plan called Sporting Future, highlighted how crucial it is to look after athletes' wellbeing and help successfully navigate their lives after retirement.[138]

While the increased recognition of support is heartening, there is still scope for further improvement, as retirement is pretty much the only inevitable outcome in any athlete's career. As illustrated by the tragic case of Jeremy Wisten, there can be a perception that when an athlete is no longer deemed essential to a club or sporting institution, they may be cast aside. Consequently, the need for transitional programmes to support the young men and women coming to the end of their careers is an increasingly vital cog in the sporting landscape.

THE SECOND ACT – FINDING PURPOSE BEYOND ATHLETIC IDENTITY

There is a degree of "natural" ability that is required to make it to the top of any sport. However, as discussed previously, most athletes still require an astonishing amount of dedication and fortitude to make it as a professional. It's easy to see how retirement can be a daunting transition for elite athletes. The physical, emotional and mental toll of rigorous training, constant competition and the pursuit of glory can consume athletes for years. Retirement marks a significant change, and the absence of the intense demands and adrenaline-filled days can have a profound impact on athletes' mental health. In an instant, a cornerstone of their personal and professional identity is stripped away. The question naturally arises: if they are no longer professional sportspeople, then who are they?

The sudden loss of an athlete's identity, the end of a career they have invested so much into, and the adjustment to "regular" life can trigger feelings of emptiness and a struggle to find purpose. Athletes may feel like forgotten members of society as they step away from the limelight they once enjoyed. The personal, social and occupational changes associated with retirement can cause distressful reactions and a need to reconstruct and adjust to a new lifestyle.[139]

Athletes often become consumed by training, competition and results, leaving little room for developing a balanced perspective on career opportunities outside of sports. This is known as tunnel vision syndrome. When retirement approaches, athletes may find themselves unprepared and unsure of where to apply their focus and dedication. The void left by the end of routine and structure, and the uncertainty of the future can contribute to mental health challenges. It is similar to what some face when leaving the armed forces. Individuals have essentially become institutionalized, and the transition to civilian life becomes a significant challenge.

Biological factors may also play a role in the mental health challenges faced by retired athletes. Exercise can boost the production of serotonin, a naturally occurring chemical compound that helps regulate mood.[140] The sudden decrease or cessation of regular serotonin release can disrupt the body's chemistry. Serotonin imbalances have been linked to depression.[141] Despite further research being needed to explore the potential impact on retired athletes, this perhaps explains why some turn to drinking, drugs and gambling to chase that same rush that sporting glory provided them.

To support former athletes in their transition to retirement and mitigate the risk of depression, various measures can be taken. Athletes should be encouraged to expand their self-identity beyond their sporting roles, exploring other interests and activities.

It is essential to recognize that athletes, despite their perceived mental toughness, are vulnerable to challenges faced in retirement. They may also be reluctant to seek help due to societal expectations discussed previously. Retirement is a challenging process for athletes at all levels of the food chain, and social support is vital in helping to navigate this transitional period and avoid post-retirement struggles. Furthermore, the impact that athletes can have on the mental health revolution does not stop the moment they retire. The halo of influence that athletes enjoy usually shines bright many years after they hang up their boots. In some cases, it never really fades at all.

FROM THE PITCH TO THE ABYSS – PAUL GASCOIGNE'S POST-RETIREMENT STRUGGLES

Hearing the name Paul Gascoigne – or his nickname, "Gazza" – resonates deeply with England football fans of my age, who remember him as one of the most talented players our country has ever produced. However, due to accusations of squandered talent and ongoing mental health struggles, Gazza is seen as a tragic figure and a cautionary tale.

Renowned for his extraordinary skill, creativity and flair, Gascoigne is arguably the most talented and enigmatic player ever produced by England. He possessed an almost unmatched ability to break through defences with his mesmerizing runs. His vision on the pitch was extraordinary, his passes impeccable and his ball control unrivalled, allowing him to navigate through tight spaces and outmanoeuvre opponents effortlessly.

But what truly set Gascoigne apart was his audacity and unpredictability. This is probably best embodied by his goal against Scotland in Euro 96. When pressed, I would probably choose this as my single favourite moment in football.

England were hosting the tournament, and I was a fresh faced 12-year-old. The intense rivalry between the two neighbours only amplified the significance of the encounter. Looking back, the England team was stacked with incredible talent. However, on the back of their failure to qualify for the World Cup in 1994, and a series of controversies surrounding an alcohol fuelled pre-tournament tour in Hong Kong – morale was not high leading into the tournament. This feeling was only amplified by a disappointing draw with Switzerland in the opening game.

Next up was Scotland. England took a second-half lead through Alan Shearer, but heading into the final quarter of the match, Scotland were awarded a penalty. David Seaman saved the spot kick, and seconds later, it happened...

The ball found its way across the pitch to Gascoigne, just outside the penalty area. With remarkable composure and instinctive brilliance, he flicked the ball over the head of Scotland defender Colin Hendry and met it perfectly on the volley with his right foot, arrowing the ball into the bottom corner of the goal.

Gascoigne, overwhelmed by the sheer magnitude of the moment, embarked on a celebration that would forever be etched in the memories of England fans. He lay flat on his back while teammate Shearer sprayed a Lucozade bottle into his mouth. It would forever be known as the "dentist chair". The original incident, a booze-soaked escapade in Hong Kong, had seen photos of Gascoigne and his teammates in various stages of alcohol-fuelled revelry splashed across the tabloids. Criticism was swift and harsh. But Gascoigne, never one to shy away from the spotlight or a chance to turn the tables on his detractors, transformed his goal celebration into a cheeky retort, a playful yet potent message to the media. It was a moment of pure Gazza: irreverent, iconic and unforgettable.

In hindsight, it was probably the high-water mark for Gascoigne. It was never that good again.

But beyond his technical brilliance, Gascoigne possessed an infectious charisma that captivated fans and teammates alike. His playful and mischievous nature endeared him to supporters, as he approached the game and life with a childlike enthusiasm and naivety.

Long before that iconic goal at Euro 96, Gascoigne burst onto the scene at the tender age of 17 when he made his league debut for his beloved local team Newcastle United in 1985. Within three years, he had already won the PFA Young Player of the Year award, a testament to his immense talent and potential. In 1988, he joined Tottenham Hotspur for a then English record transfer fee of £2.3 million, further cementing his rise to stardom.

It was during the 1990 World Cup that Gascoigne rose to household fame. It also revealed his fragility and vulnerability that won him the love of the nation. Following a yellow card in the semi-final against West Germany, which ruled him out of a potential appearance in the final, Gazza could not hold back his tears of frustration. Despite England's subsequent defeat on penalties, Gascoigne's on-field displays and raw emotion earned him the BBC Sports Personality of the Year and endeared him to the nation.

However, Gascoigne's career soon began to encounter obstacles. In the 1991 FA Cup final, he suffered a severe cruciate ligament injury that delayed his transfer to SS Lazio, a club based in Rome. Although he eventually completed the move to Italy, Gascoigne was never quite the same again.

In 1995, he returned to the UK to join Rangers, quickly gaining cult hero status on the blue side of Glasgow. The following year he was a key player in the England team during Euro 96, before once again losing in a semi-final to Germany.

As talented as he was, Gascoigne was equally tormented off the pitch. A combination of factors, including injuries, substance abuse and the pressures of fame, weighed heavily on him. It was around this time that Gascoigne's personal life began to unravel, with incidents of domestic violence and alcoholism leading to the end of his marriage.

Throughout the late 1990s and early 2000s, Gascoigne's struggles with mental health issues and addiction gained significant public attention. His battle with obsessive-compulsive disorder, bulimia and depression were brought to the forefront. But it was his battle with alcoholism that resulted in him being a mainstay of the tabloid press.

Gascoigne struggled throughout his career. However, it wasn't until he finally retired as a professional, in low-key circumstances at Boston United in 2004, that things really seemed to fall apart. Without football to give him a reason to stay fit and sober, alcoholism fully gripped him, and his physical appearance notably declined.

Gascoigne's erratic behaviour culminated in his involvement in the Raoul Moat incident in 2010. Moat instantly became a notorious figure in the UK when, on 3 July of that year, he went on a shooting spree, wounding his ex-girlfriend, killing her new boyfriend and blinding a police officer. Eventually, police were able to chase down the gunman and corner him in a stand-off – and that's when Gascoigne arrived.

The former football star showed up at the scene claiming to be a friend of Moat's and attempting to broker peace between the armed police and the fugitive gunman. But this wasn't true, thus highlighting the fragility of Gascoigne's mental state at the time, and his need for professional help and support.

The road to recovery has been a tumultuous one for Gascoigne. He has sought treatment on multiple occasions, including admissions to clinics and rehab centres. His struggles with alcoholism and the consequences of his actions have resulted in legal issues and strained relationships.

The tragedy in Paul Gascoigne's life lies in his deep need for love and support, a vulnerability that made him an easy target for exploitation. His story exemplifies the importance of a robust support network, one that could have guided him toward a healthier path and protected him from those who exploited his talent and resources.

Although they appear very different, I believe there is a great deal that united Gazza and Mike Tyson, two men who had too much, too fast. They had nobody around to have the hard conversations with and keep them on the right path. Perhaps this kind of behaviour occurs among those who are the most gifted. Perhaps it is because everything came that much easier for them in the first place.

However, when the dust settles at the end of a career, and the crowd of followers thins out as fame and fortune dwindle, it's especially sad. Despite his controversies, Gascoigne deserves empathy and understanding. His story highlights how important it is to take care of our mental health. It should make us question the role of the tabloid media in exploiting the struggles of those in the spotlight. It also calls for us, the audience who consumes these stories, to consider the impact on the lives of those who bear the weight of fame.

At the core of the mental health revolution is the crucial need to offer more empathy to individuals who face challenges while living in the public eye. Celebrities, athletes and public figures often endure immense pressure and scrutiny, which can significantly impact their mental wellbeing. Instead of looking down on them, showing a bit of kindness and support can make a big difference. This shift toward being more understanding and caring is a big step in changing how we think about mental health. It's all about treating everyone with compassion, no matter who they are. By pushing for a world where empathy is key, we're working toward a place where taking care of your mental health is normal, and people can get help without worrying about being judged.

FINDING BALANCE – IAN THORPE'S COPING STRATEGIES IN RETIREMENT

Ian Thorpe is an Australian swimming legend who retired at the age of 24. He achieved incredible success during his career, shattering 22 world records and amassing a collection of Olympic medals: five gold, three silver and one bronze. However, behind his exceptional achievements lay a lifelong battle with depression and other mental health issues that started during his teenage years.

Being in the public spotlight compounded Thorpe's struggles at times. The constant reminders of his remarkable athletic accomplishments often left him questioning why he felt the way he did. He admitted, "It becomes difficult when you try to rationalize that. There's also a sense of guilt for not feeling on top of the world when really you should be. But if you're a depressed person in a depressed state, you don't rationalize things well."[142]

This raises some important questions. Why do we equate success with happiness? Are we prone to assuming that individuals clutching trophies must be elated? Thorpe's case seems to suggest otherwise. As with the previous examples of Marcus Trescothick and Tyson Fury, their biggest mental health emergencies came in the immediate aftermath of some of their greatest career achievements. We naturally place value on achieving goals and reaching milestones. It's easy to think that when you get to a certain point in your career, you'll be happy, or when you achieve a goal, it will make you content. But it's the process along the way to any of those things, that's where the real happiness is. And if you don't find it, you're never going to be fulfilled when you get there.

As we have been exploring in this chapter, one of the core challenges for elite athletes is navigating the transition to life after sports. For Thorpe, this involved shifting his focus from one form of champion to another. He dedicated himself to causes such as mental health, Indigenous literacy and LGBTQI+ rights.

Thorpe has delved into the subject of career transitions for former top-level athletes. He agrees that a lot of athletes base their self-worth only on their status as sportspeople and don't work on other parts of their lives. Reflecting on his own transition to retirement, Thorpe admits that he always thought of himself as more than whatever he did in the pool. He had a mindset that he still wanted to do great things with the rest of his life.[143]

Many athletes have spoken out about their struggles with depression, but Thorpe's story stands out to me. He's been incredibly open about how he deals with depression every day, especially after retiring. By sharing his experiences, he offers useful tips on how to cope with depression, helping others who are going through similar challenges.

Acceptance forms the cornerstone of Thorpe's practice. As an athlete driven to be the best, he grappled with the notion of not being able to handle the challenges of everyday life. This internal struggle persisted throughout his sporting career, and especially after retirement.[144] However, he eventually had an epiphany that changed his perspective entirely. Thorpe acknowledged the importance of embracing his vulnerability and understanding that perfection was not a prerequisite for a good life. By gaining a deeper understanding of himself and implementing coping strategies, he found that his life improved significantly.

A cornerstone of his recovery is the philosophy of granting oneself a day off every now and then. He has learned the importance of acknowledging that some days will not be his best, and on those days, he allows himself to take a break. He sets clear boundaries, designating one day for rest, knowing that the following day he will be able to resume his usual activities. Dismissing these moments of struggle would only add to the burden he already carries, so he chooses to acknowledge and honour his need for respite.

Another key way he's managed to cope is through his circle of support. Throughout this book, we've seen stories of athletes who didn't have enough reliable people around them. For Thorpe, having a tight-knit group has been a game-changer. He has learned how important it is to talk about what he's going through, and to reach out for help when necessary. But getting to this point wasn't easy. At first, he was reluctant to share his struggles with those closest to him, not wanting to burden his family during his younger years.

Reflecting on this, Thorpe later recognized that his loved ones would have done anything to support him. He emphasizes the importance of understanding that those struggling with mental health problems often lack rational thinking and are unaware of the abundance of support available to them. Fortunately, Thorpe was able to confide in friends, colleagues and mentors, all of whom provided him guidance and assistance.

This is something that struck a chord with me. It's common for many of us to assume that people wouldn't want to be burdened with our struggles. However, the reality is that most of us have at least a few individuals who would always be there, offering support during our most challenging moments, if only they were aware of our needs.

I think there are key takeaways from Ian Thorpe's personal journey that can apply to anyone's life. By accepting vulnerability, acknowledging the issue, granting oneself time off when necessary and building a reliable support network, most people can at least alleviate the stresses and strains they may be suffering in their own lives. These insights from Thorpe could very well be the framework of or manifesto for the mental health revolution.

Like many athletes, Thorpe struggled with the dramatic life transition that occurs during retirement. As he put it, "You go from doing between 30 and 40 hours of training a week, to then wanting not only to fill in that time, but also find something you're passionate about again."[145] Maybe the real challenge with retiring from sports is the expectation that comes with it. Being incredibly successful in one area, like sports, is rare in itself. Yet, many athletes expect to replicate this success in another phase of their lives after retirement. This expectation can add an extra layer of pressure, as transitioning from an elite sporting career to a different role or identity isn't straightforward. Athletes often dedicate their entire lives to perfecting their skills in their sport, and when it's time to move on, finding a new passion or career that brings similar levels of success and fulfilment can be a daunting task. This transition requires not just adapting to a new lifestyle, but also redefining one's sense of purpose and identity outside of the sports arena.

LURKING MENTAL HEALTH ISSUES

An athlete's retirement can induce a profound identity crisis that can consume them when they reach the end of their professional career. As we saw with the examples of Gascoigne, Bruno and Thorpe, there are also those who have pre-existing mental health challenges, which the routine, safety and fringe benefits of exercise can help alleviate for a time. When they retire, those problems do not go away. If anything, there is the danger and possibility that they are intensified.

For most athletes, their glory days are fleeting, and they find themselves retiring at a relatively young age with a considerable proportion of their lives still ahead. The decision to retire from sport is no easy task. It involves bidding farewell to years of rigorous strength training, physical conditioning and intense competition. It means leaving behind the roar of crowds, the cheers from devoted fans and the affirmations from coaches and teammates. While retirement doesn't necessarily imply the end of work for elite athletes, it entails a complete lifestyle change. Adjusting to this transition requires an immense amount of adaptation.

While most athletes retire at a young age, they also usually begin their sporting journeys during their formative years. An elite sportsperson, driven by their passion for their chosen sport, dedicates countless hours to honing their skills and athletic abilities while juggling the demands of regular life. Their sport isn't just something they do – it becomes a huge part of who they are. So, when it's time to hang up their boots and move on, it's not just a career change. Instead, it feels like they're leaving a piece of themselves behind. This transition is tough because their sport has shaped so much of their life and identity.

Athletes are not solely defined by their physical abilities – they possess a multitude of personal traits and characteristics. However, this fact is sometimes forgotten, even by the athletes themselves. It is crucial for athletes to recognize their individuality beyond their sporting prowess. Engaging in regular self-care strategies and exploring other talents, hobbies and interests can help alleviate the feeling of being completely lost after retirement.

It is also important to not solely look at this through the lens of the most highly paid athletes in the world. The majority of professional sportspeople will not make enough money during their career to sustain themselves and their families for the rest of their lives. As such, many will *need* to pivot their lives and find employment after sport. This in and of itself can help with ensuring their lives remain purposeful. However, for all athletes that come to the end of their careers, planning and preparation is a must. As Serena Williams eloquently put it, "I'm evolving away from tennis, toward other things that are important to me."[146]

10

THE IMPORTANCE OF BEING YOURSELF

The Key to Thriving as a Professional Athlete

Maslow's Hierarchy of Needs is a highly influential theory proposed by the American psychologist Abraham Maslow, first published in 1943. It suggests that humans have a set of needs that must be fulfilled in a specific order to achieve their full potential. Maslow proposed that as each need is met, individuals are motivated to pursue the next level, leading to the ultimate goal of self-fulfilment.

The hierarchy is usually depicted as a pyramid with five distinct levels, arranged from the most basic to the highest. The foundational level of the pyramid is "physiological needs", and represents the most essential requirements for survival, such as food, water, shelter and sleep. These needs must be satisfied before an individual can focus on higher levels of the pyramid.

Once physiological needs are met, individuals seek the level of "safety and security". This includes personal and financial stability, protection from harm and a safe environment. Examples of safety needs include job security, access to healthcare, a stable living environment and protection from violence or threats.

After satisfying the safety needs, the next level on the hierarchy relates to "love and belongingness". People strive for a sense of love, belonging and social connection. This includes forming meaningful relationships, friendships, and a sense of acceptance and belonging within a community or group. One could argue that this level of the pyramid is exactly the reason why we form communities around sports teams in the first place.

Next up are "esteem-based needs", which refer to the desire for self-esteem, self-respect and recognition from others. This includes both internal factors, such as self-confidence, competence and achievements, as well as external factors, like social status, reputation and respect from others. Fulfilling these needs helps individuals develop a positive self-image and a sense of accomplishment.

At the very top of the hierarchy is "self-actualization", which represents the fulfilment of an individual's highest potential and the pursuit of personal growth. Self-actualization involves the realization of one's talents, creativity, potential and the ability to become the best version of oneself. It is characterized by a strong desire for personal development, self-fulfilment and a deep sense of purpose.

In this next section, I am going to explore some examples of athletes who were denied access to the upper echelons of the Maslow pyramid. Then, I will examine the consequences it had on their careers, mental health and ability to reach their full potential.

JUSTIN AND JAKE

Thankfully, attitudes toward the LGBTQI+ community have changed radically in my lifetime. This journey is perhaps best exemplified by the parallel lives of Justin Fashanu and Jake Daniels.

Fashanu became the first openly gay player in English football in 1990, and it would be 32 years before another player followed suit. In 2022, 17-year-old Blackpool FC forward Jake Daniels took the decision to go public about his sexuality. Jake's motivation for this move stemmed from his unwavering commitment to authenticity. He chose to be open with the world about his sexuality just days after coming out to his family. After the conversation with his loved ones, he played in a youth fixture against Accrington Stanley, in which he scored four goals. He admitted, "It just shows how much of a weight off the shoulders it was."[147]

It is both noteworthy and incredibly sad that there was a 32-year gap between the first and second out and active male professional footballers in England. The female game has had much less of a problem with homophobia, but in men's football, it remains a significant problem and trails far behind the progress that has been made in wider society, despite the best efforts of LGBTQI+ fan groups that represent clubs up and down the country.

As of 2024, there are currently more than 5,000 male professional footballers in England.[148] The average footballing career is about eight years.[149] And around 3 per cent of men in the general population in the UK identify as gay.[150] Even accounting for a hyper-masculine skew in football that may be off-putting for potential gay players, it feels like a statistical impossibility that, in the 32 years between Fashanu and Daniels, none of the thousands of footballers who laced up their boots were gay, too. In fact, we know this is true, as German international Thomas Hitzlsperger, who played for West Ham, Aston Villa and Everton, came out after retirement.

Sadly, given some of the less-than-enlightened views that still come from the terraces at football stadiums today, I do not blame any gay professional footballers who take the decision to remain in the closet.

Justin Fashanu is a potent example of a man who surely would have benefited from living in another, more open-minded era. He was a man who was frequently denied the ability to achieve "self-actualization". As a result, he never achieved his full potential, and his life was ultimately cut tragically short.

Fashanu began his career in the late 1970s for Norwich City, his local club. At Norwich he delivered a string of eye-catching performances, including a goal against reigning First Division champions Liverpool, which won him the BBC Goal of the Season award.

Fashanu was then called up to the England under-21 team, scoring five goals in 11 appearances. It seemed he was destined for greatness. With Fashanu's enormous potential, it came as little surprise when he became the first Black player to command a £1 million transfer fee, when he signed for Nottingham Forest and their legendary if uncompromising coach, Brian Clough.

Nottingham Forest may not be the biggest draw in English football today, but when Fashanu joined, they had just won back-to-back European Cups, now known as the Champions League. His move represented the hottest young talent in the country joining an already formidable team, with the greatest coach of his generation at the helm. It should have been a match made in heaven. To say it went badly wrong is an understatement. His career at Forest was a disaster – he scored just three times in 33 games.

Brian Clough remains to this day a footballing icon, a larger-than-life figure whose charisma and uncompromising style made him one of the most memorable managers in the history of the game. His impact on English football was immense, and his legacy endures to this day.

But Clough was a complex character, a man who could be both charming and abrasive, often at the same time. He was a masterful motivator, able to inspire his players to greatness with a few well-chosen words, but he was also capable of berating them in public if he felt they weren't performing up to his standards.

Perhaps Clough's crowning glory were the aforementioned back-to-back European Cups with Forest. This was a remarkable achievement for a club that had been languishing in the Second Division just a few years earlier, and it was partly driven by Clough's sheer force of personality. He was also not afraid to make tough decisions. He famously sold his star striker Trevor Francis to Manchester City in 1981, despite the protests of Forest fans.

Clough's success at Forest was all the more remarkable given his fractious relationship with the club's board. He was a man who spoke his mind and wasn't afraid to take on authority, and this often led to clashes with the people in charge. But he was always able to win them over with his results on the pitch; his achievements at Forest stand alone as an outlier, not just for the club, but in European football as a whole. Even after suffering relegation with the club during a very public battle with alcoholism, the fans still adored him, and they continue to sing his name to this very day.

I had always held Clough on a pedestal as a charming and charismatic man who couldn't beat his demons. Undoubtedly, in his pomp, he ranks among the greatest managers the game has ever seen. However, it was only upon researching for this book that I realized the central role that Clough played in Justin Fashanu's downfall.

Partly due to Fashanu's poor goal return, Forest and Clough quickly regretted the transfer. Clough then heard through the grapevine of Fashanu's visits to local gay bars in the city.

Upon discovering Fashanu was gay, Clough barred him from training with the first team, an act of intolerance that feels barely believable when viewed through the prism of modern values. Later reflecting on what had happened, Clough seemingly felt little remorse for his actions. He wrote in his autobiography that he once derided Fashanu in a meeting, asking Fashanu in front of his teammates, "Where do you go if you want a loaf of bread? A baker's, I suppose. Where do you go if you want a leg of lamb? A butcher. So why do you keep going to that bloody poofs' club?"[151]

It's little wonder that Fashanu struggled on the pitch. An enormous price tag is enough of a burden for many players, let alone the almost unimaginable stress of your boss despising you for who you are. Now, imagine that boss having near king-like status in your work environment – how could Fashanu possibly thrive? As Dr Pippa Grange asserts, "None of these overtly controlling, fear-based environments are places where you can bud, then blossom."[152]

After Forest, the remainder of Fashanu's career resembled that of a nomadic journeyman. He never hit the heights that his early career had suggested possible. He rarely stayed in one place for more than a few seasons at a time, slowly slipping down the leagues and picking up pay checks in footballing outposts such as (pre-Major League Soccer) USA, Canada and New Zealand. It was an almost unimaginable fate for the red-hot prospect for whom Forest stumped up a record fee.

It wasn't until nearly a decade after that initial move to Nottingham Forest that Justin Fashanu came out publicly. In October 1990, in need of cash, he agreed to an exclusive with *The Sun* newspaper, who ran the headline, "£1m Football Star: I AM GAY". The article also made claims about an affair with a Conservative Member of Parliament, something that Fashanu himself later said was fabricated by the newspaper.[153]

The article was essentially the final nail in the coffin of Fashanu's career at the highest level. It was also the catalyst behind the very public fracturing of the relationship between Justin and his older brother John, who tried to pay him £75,000 not to release the story. John also gave a story to *The Voice* a week after the article, in which he called Justin the outcast of the family. John later admitted that he regretted his behaviour during that time. Nevertheless, despite John's admission, the brothers never managed to reconcile.

In March 1998, while working as a coach for Maryland Mania in the US, Fashanu was accused of sexually assaulting a 17-year-old. Homosexual acts were illegal in Maryland at the time, and being Black, Fashanu feared he would be unlikely to get a fair trial. He fled the US returning to England.

On 3 May 1998, Justin Fashanu, the first Black million-pound footballer, was found dead in a garage he had broken into in Shoreditch, East London, after visiting Chariots, a local gay sauna. In his suicide note, he denied the charges, claiming the sex was consensual, but his lack of faith in the US judicial system had driven him to take his own life.

It is impossible to say what Justin Fashanu could have achieved if he'd had a loving support network around him. A manager that didn't ostracize him for his sexuality. A brother who didn't abandon him when he needed him most. Who knows how far he could have gone?

We live in a far from perfect world, yet I am genuinely thankful that Jake Daniels will not have to endure the institutional bigotry that plagued Justin Fashanu through his short and turbulent life.

With the progress that is being made societally on the issue of homophobia, it seems a reasonable bet that it will not take another 32 years for the next professional footballer in England to come out as gay. In fact, during the process of writing this book, Jakub Jankto, the Cagliari Calcio and Czech Republic international, has done just that, becoming the most high-profile active gay player to date.

However, in many ways, the speed of this change relies as much on the behaviour of fans and coaches as it does the bravery of players to come out in the first place. Creating an inclusive atmosphere in which gay players are not singled out for abuse is crucial to embolden others to follow in the footsteps of Daniels and Jankto. Who knows, in 32 more years, we may be in a position where a footballer coming out as gay is met with a shrug, or better still, a complete lack of interest.

Likewise, I would suggest that we want as many athletes as possible to ascend to the very top of Maslow's Hierarchy of Needs. By reaching the top of the pyramid, they will be more likely to fulfil their potential. This, however, necessitates creating an environment where they feel comfortable with all aspects of who they are. This naturally includes any mental health issues they may be suffering. In the same way that Justin Fashanu had to hide so much of himself, meaning he was never able to flourish and achieve self-actualization, then surely the same is true of those who suppress their diagnosable mental health issues. Creating an environment where the majority of sportspeople are comfortable revealing and discussing mental health episodes could actually be a net positive to overall performance within the athletic community. I believe that, through some of the first mental health pioneers that we have discussed in this book, that process is already well under way. The wheels are in motion. How quickly we get to that inevitable end point is largely down to the environment that sports administrators and coaches create, as well as how we as a society embrace the oncoming mental health revolution.

CONCLUSION

THE FUTURE

I, like many others, oscillate between hope and despair at the current state of the world. Perhaps it was always thus.

Throughout the course of the research for this book, I spoke with numerous mental health specialists. It is largely agreed that we have made a significant amount of progress on mental health issues, both societally and among the next generation of sporting talent. Yet, there is also a general acceptance among this group that toxic masculinity remains a barrier for much greater progress. Sarah Nightingale, who largely works with age-group football players, admitted, "The big thing still in sport is masculinity, that you don't want to admit weakness, in case the coach isn't going to select you."[154]

The fear of showing any form of weakness, driven by the perceived advantage you may be giving away, be it to your opponent or a rival for your spot in the team, is perhaps the single-biggest barrier to the mental health revolution, but one I genuinely believe that will be eroded away. And yet, there is seemingly only one way in which that erosion can take place: through the example of others. The history of mental health and sport is one that has arced from a period of misunderstanding and ridicule, through to an era of much greater acceptance and compassion. The next phase, being driven by the bravery of the likes of those we have discussed in this book, will help to usher in an unprecedented level of acceptance of diversity of mental health within sport. That will, in turn, be a catalyst for much greater acceptance societally.

Previously, I mentioned that sport was a powerful force in pushing greater racial equality in the West. I believe that it has a similar power to force through greater acceptance and understanding of mental health issues. To go back to the quote from Simon Barnes reflecting on Barack Obama becoming President of the United States, "Sport not only reflects society, but it is also a significant force in changing it... Sometimes Blacks are better than whites, and no one can duck that truth."[155] Also, sometimes people with acute mental health issues are better than people who don't have them. There is no ducking that truth, either.

The status we hold for our sporting icons is reserved for those at the very apex of society. They are very much alphas of national and global communities. This is why I maintain their fundamental importance in driving forward the mental health revolution. The ground has been laid. Our first protagonists have entered the stage. The progress from here on out will be exponential, not linear.

The rise in the conversation around mental health issues is actually one of the things that gives me something to be hopeful about. It's a topic that has gained considerable traction in society over the past few years, and rightly so. From being something that was swept under the carpet, mental health has emerged as a topic of discussion that is no longer relegated to the shadows.

It's been a long hard road to get here, with many unnecessary casualties along the way. At the turn of the millennium, mental health was a topic that was largely ignored. It was viewed as a weakness and something to be ashamed of. Mental illness was often stigmatized, and those who suffered from it were ostracized or simply misunderstood. The prevailing attitude was one of ignorance and fear.

As we entered the 2010s, the conversation around mental wellness began to gain mainstream momentum. Celebrities began to speak out about their struggles. The media began to cover mental health more frequently and empathetically.

This momentum is leading to a generational shift in attitudes. Among younger people, there is a greater understanding of the importance of mental wellbeing, and the impact that it has on our daily lives. There are reams of evidence that Generation Z are more open about their mental health than any previous generation. According to a survey conducted by the American Psychological Association, 91 per cent of Gen Z adults said that they felt comfortable talking about their mental health, compared to just 73 per cent of baby boomers.[156]

Also, Gen Z are nearly three times more likely to have seen a therapist since the pandemic than baby boomers.[157]

Facts and figures like these can be erroneously massaged by those who have an agenda against progressive values. This group often targets Gen Z and their openness as a weakness. I happen to think the opposite. Being increasingly honest about our mental health is not the symptom of more problems in society; it is the very bedrock and foundation of the mental health revolution.

There has been a significant increase in the diagnosis of mental health conditions over recent decades, not just in the UK and the West, but also globally. This may suggest that the stresses and pressures of modern life, including factors we are now only just getting to grips with, may be driving a mental health crisis. It may be possible that social media, fake news and unlimited internet access may be exacerbating mental health problems. However, if we take the UK as a stand-alone example, the rate of death by suicide in 1990 was around 13 in every 100,000 people; at the time of writing this book, the rate is around 11 in 100,000.[158] I don't want to trivialize these statistics, as I have a friend and a family member who both died by suicide. I know how painful it is to lose someone this way. Yet, the raw evidence suggests that this is something that is becoming less common as we open ourselves up to our own vulnerability. It stands to reason that through greater awareness and recognition of mental health problems, people are more likely to seek help and receive a diagnosis.

Not only are Gen Z more open toward issues surrounding mental health, but there is evidence they are more understanding of intersectionality of others in general. According to a recent report, 57 per cent of Gen Z-ers believe that increasing racial and ethnic diversity is good for society, compared to 42 per cent of baby boomers.[159] Also, a report by the LGTBQ advocacy organization GLAAD found that 20 per cent of Gen Z-ers identify as LGBTQ, compared to just 2 per cent of baby boomers.[160] I find it impossible to believe that there are ten times more gay people now than 50 years ago. Instead, I believe we have a generation of people who are much more likely to embrace who they are, something I also happen to believe comes with significant mental health benefits.

Yet, I also know we do not live in a utopian fantasy. Reports of homophobic hate crimes have more than doubled in five years, rising from 10,000 in 2017 to nearly 27,000 in 2022.[161] I believe that this shocking rise in hate crimes is at least partly driven by right-wing rhetoric, deployed in the culture wars to target LGBTQI+ groups. However fanatical those voices are, the reality is they are also becoming increasingly fringe and opposed with modern Western values. The progress that has been made in recent years does nothing to assuage me of that belief. The arc of history bends toward justice, and we must stay on this path.

SCRATCHING THE SURFACE

When I set out to write this book, I did so in the belief that we had made significant ground in relation to our understanding and empathy toward issues of mental health. In many ways, I still believe that. After all, we don't have to look back too far in history to find examples where athletes have been mistreated in ways that would seem unimaginable today.

Yet, we are still very much in the embryonic stages of the mental health revolution. There is still so much progress to be made. Michio Kaku, a theoretical physicist, points out that the human brain is the most complex thing in the known universe, with "100 billion neurons each connected to 10,000 others."[162] As long as humans have existed, people have sought to and failed to fully comprehend our most powerful tool. We may also feel like we live in an age of unprecedented technological progress. However, this sentiment is not unique to our time. In 1900, Lord Kelvin, a British mathematician, boldly claimed that "there is nothing new to be discovered in physics now. All that remains is more and more precise measurement."[163] Looking ahead, if humanity endures for another century and a quarter, the potential for astonishing scientific breakthroughs is immense.

If anything, the rate of progress will only increase ever faster. In his 1999 book *The Age of Spiritual Machines*, Ray Kurzweil proposed something that he called the "Law of Accelerating Returns". It simply means that the rate of change in a wide variety of evolutionary systems tends to increase exponentially. An analysis of the history of tech shows that this is true, contrary to the common-sense, "intuitive linear" view that things progress more gradually. His argument proposes that we won't experience 100 years of progress in the 21st century – it will be more like 20,000 years have passed.[164] This speed of progress allows us to unlock even the deepest and most complicated mysteries of the universe, including those contained within our brains.

Unless we see some huge breakthroughs in anti-aging and manage to dodge the worst outcomes of climate change, I won't be here to witness the end of the 21st century. However, I'm hopeful that with more advanced technology and a society that's becoming more open, we'll increasingly understand and care for athletes' mental health better. This will mean scrutinizing everything, from their diet and recovery through to the pressures they face from various sources, through the lens of mental wellbeing. In simple terms, it will be a mental health revolution in sport.

However, I also believe that, fundamentally, as humans, we are hardwired to be affected by the power of stories. As such, the most crucial part of our advancement on the issue will always be on the shoulders of athletes, such as the ones who I have referenced in this book. Their bravery and openness have the power to move the narrative forward in the most profound way possible.

Sport has a strange grip over us. We would be foolish to underestimate its power.

ACKNOWLEDGEMENTS

This book is dedicated to my wonderful wife, Teresa Ferreira. It is no exaggeration to say that without your unwavering belief and support, this book would simply not exist. Everyone needs someone like Teresa in their life.

In addition, I am profoundly grateful to my family. Thank you for creating a nurturing environment where I was encouraged to question, to explore and to be rebellious, whilst always knowing I was deeply loved and supported.

I must also extend a special thank you to Beth Bishop and the entire team at Trigger Publishing for taking a chance on an unknown author. Your willingness to embrace new voices and stories is more important than ever.

FURTHER RESOURCES

BOOKS

- *Fear Less: How to Win at Life Without Losing Yourself* – Dr Pippa Grange
- *Black Box Thinking: The Surprising Truth About Success* – Matthew Syed
- *Bounce: The of Myth of Talent and the Power of Practice* – Matthew Syed
- *This Ragged Grace: A Memoir of Recovery and Renewal* – Octavia Bright
- *Outliers: The Story of Success* – Malcolm Gladwell
- *Concussed: Sport's Uncomfortable Truth* – Sam Peters
- *Unforgettable* – Steve Thompson
- *Get Your Head in the Game: An Exploration of Football's Complicated Relationship with Mental Health* – Dominic Stevenson
- *Thinking, Fast and Slow* – Daniel Kahneman
- *The Greatest: What Sport Teaches Us About Achieving Success* – Matthew Syed
- *The Sports Gene: Talent, Practice and the Truth About Success* – David Epstein
- *Range: Why Generalists Triumph in a Specialized World* – David Epstein
- *Stranger Than We Can Imagine: Making Sense of the Twentieth Century* – John Higgs
- *The Age of Spiritual Machines: When Computers Exceed Human Intelligence* – Ray Kurzweil

- *Flow: The Psychology of Optimal Experience* – Mihaly Csikszentmihalyi
- *Undisputed Truth: My Autobiography* – Mike Tyson
- *Coming Back to Me* – Marcus Trescothick
- *Sapiens: A Brief History of Humankind* – Yuval Noah Harari
- *Born to Run: The Hidden Tribe, the Ultra-Runners, and the Greatest Race the World Has Never Seen* – Christopher McDougall

DOCUMENTARIES AND TV SERIES

- *Ronnie O'Sullivan: The Edge of Everything*
- *Mark Cavendish: Never Enough*
- *Dark Side of the Ring*
- *Tour de France: Unchained*
- *Untold: Johnny Football*
- *Bruno v Tyson*
- *At Home with The Furys*

PODCASTS

- *Elis James and John Robins*
- *How Do You Cope?*
- *Football Weekly*
- *Radiolab*
- *Revisionist History*
- *Science Vs*

REFERENCES

1 Sayid, Ruki. (7 June 2012). Tear we go: Men cry more at footie than the birth of their first child. *The Mirror*. https://www.mirror.co.uk/news/uk-news/men-cry-more-at-football-than-the-birth-864707

2 *Forbes India*. (1 April 2024). The 10 most followed Instagram accounts in the world in 2024. https://www.forbesindia.com/article/explainers/most-followed-instagram-accounts-world/85649/1

3 Rech, Dominic. (11 October 2018). World Mental Health Day: Ex-footballer pushes for a 'mental health revolution' after multiple suicide attempts. CNN. https://edition.cnn.com/2018/10/10/sport/world-mental-health-day-suicide-depression-clarke-carlisle-spt-intl/index.html

4 World Health Organization. (2011). Suicide. https://www.who.int/news-room/fact-sheets/detail/suicide

5 Barnes, Simon. (2010). *Bounce: The Myth of Talent and the Power of Practice,* p259. HarperCollins UK: London.

6 Badenhausen, Kurt. (3 May 2020) Michael Jordan Has Made Over $1 Billion From Nike — The Biggest Endorsement Bargain In Sports. *Forbes*. https://www.forbes.com/sites/kurtbadenhausen/2020/05/03/michael-jordans-1-billion-nike-endorsement-is-the-biggest-bargain-in-sports/

7 Barna, George. (10 April 2013). Athletes Influence Greater than Faith Leaders. https://www.barna.com/research/athletes-influence-greater-than-faith-leaders/

8 Trescothick, Marcus and Harman, Jo. (26 August 2019). Marcus Trescothick: 'One knock changed my career.' *Wisden*. https://wisden.com/stories/magazine/marcus-trescothick-one-knock-changed-my-career

9 McRae, Donald. (21 June 2011). Marcus Trescothick: Depression and me. *The Guardian*. https://www.theguardian.com/sport/2011/jun/21/marcus-trescothick-interview

10 Fury, Tyson. (October 2018). *The Joe Rogan Experience*. https://www.youtube.com/watch?v=XrM6WqYEj9Y

11 Ingle, Sean. (23 February 2020). Tyson Fury: from the lowest of lows to the top of the world. *The Guardian*. https://www.theguardian.com/sport/2020/feb/23/tyson-fury-heavyweight-boxing-highs-lows

12 Beirne, Kevin. (5 December 2018). 'Tyson Fury's sexist and homophobic remarks would make him the most undeserving BBC Sports Personality of the Year ever.' *The Independent*. https://www.independent.co.uk/voices/tyson-fury-deontay-wilder-bbc-sports-personality-year-2019-racism-homophobia-antisemitism-a8668091.html

13 Lehman, Jonathan. (4 December 2015). Boxing champ: 'A woman's best place is on her back'. *New York Post.* https://nypost.com/2015/12/04/boxing-champ-a-womans-best-place-is-on-her-back/

14 Sweeney, Sarah, and Dolling, Billie. (21 August 2020). A research paper: Suicide Prevention in Traveller communities in England. https://www.gypsy-traveller.org/wp-content/uploads/2020/10/Suicide-Prevention-Report-FINAL.pdf

15 The Traveller Movement. (March 2019). The Traveller Movement – policy briefing addressing mental health and suicide among Gypsy, Roma and Traveller communities in England. https://wp-main.travellermovement.org.uk/wp-content/uploads/2021/09/Mental-Health-and-Suicide-among-GRT-communities-in-England-Briefing-2019.pdf

16 Mayo Clinic. (2017). Depression and anxiety: Exercise eases symptoms. https://www.mayoclinic.org/diseases-conditions/depression-and-exercise/art-20046495

17 Gage, Fred. (31 January 2011). Exercise training increases size of hippocampus and improves memory. https://www.ncbi.nlm.nih.gov/pmc/articles/PMC3041121/

18 O'Sullivan, Ronnie. (2023). *Desert Island Discs.* BBC. https://www.bbc.co.uk/programmes/m001mc30

19 Ericsson, K. Anders, and Krampe, Ralf Th. (July 1993). The Role of Deliberate Practice in the Acquisition of Expert Performance. *Psychological Review.* https://www.colorado.edu/ics/sites/default/files/attached-files/91-06.pdf

20 Miller, Michael. (20 June 2022). The Great Practice Myth: Debunking the 10,000 Hour Rule. https://www.6seconds.org/2022/06/20/10000-hour-rule/

21 Syed, Matthew. (April 2011). *Bounce: The of Myth of Talent and the Power of Practice*. Fourth Estate.

22 Epstein, David. (January 2014). *The Sports Gene: Talent, Practice and the Truth About Success.* Yellow Jersey.

23 Damjanovic, Jelena. (30 July 2021). Elite athletes more likely to experience mental health disorders: U of T study. https://www.kpe.utoronto.ca/faculty-news/elite-athletes-more-likely-experience-mental-health-disorders-u-t-study

24 Ibid.

25 Epstein, David. (January 2014). *The Sports Gene: Talent, Practice and the Truth About Success.* Yellow Jersey.

26 Ibid.

27 Philips, Stephen. (11 August 2017). The Average Guy Who Spent 6,003 Hours Trying to Be a Professional Golfer. *The Atlantic.* https://www.theatlantic.com/health/archive/2017/08/the-dan-plan/536592/

28 Epstein, David. (January 2014). *The Sports Gene: Talent, Practice and the Truth About Success.* Yellow Jersey.

29 Sussman, Oliver. (9 November 2023). Diathesis–Stress Model. https://www.simplypsychology.org/diathesis-stress-model.html#:~:text=According%20to%20the%20diathesis%2Dstress,the%20development%20of%20the%20disorder

30 Cooks-Campbell, Allaya. (4 February 2022). Mental health in athletes: Physical prowess, mental fitness. https://www.betterup.com/blog/mental-health-in-athletes

31 Cleveland Clinic. (10 August 2021). Athletes and Mental Health: Breaking the Stigma. https://health.clevelandclinic.org/mental-health-in-athletes/

32 Trine University. (21 June 2022). Prioritizing Mental Health in College Athletes. https://www.trine.edu/academics/centers/center-for-sports-studies/blog/2022/prioritizing_mental_health_in_college_athletes.aspx

33 AZ Quotes. Randall "Tex" Cobb Quotes. https://www.azquotes.com/quote/553179

34 Free Think. (22 April 2022). Inside the boxing gym that trains kids for life, not to fight. https://www.freethink.com/series/catalysts/fighting-poverty

35 Tyson, Mike. (2013). *Undisputed Truth*. HarperSport.

36 Cancian, Dan. (25 May 2021). What Did Mike Tyson and Robin Givens Say in Barbara Walters Interview? *Newsweek*. https://www.newsweek.com/mike-tyson-robin-givens-barbara-walters-interview-1594178

37 BLTV Classic. (2 April 2022). Mike Was Terrifying on Pro Debut! https://www.youtube.com/watch?v=HENlNxtlQ0E

38 Smith, Nick. (14 November 2023). Mike Tyson's Undisputed Truth – the book's 10 most astonishing claims. *The Guardian*. https://www.theguardian.com/sport/2013/nov/14/mike-tyson-undisputed-truth-astonishing-claims

39 University of Rochester Medical Center. (1 May 2024). How Childhood Trauma May Impact Adults. https://www.urmc.rochester.edu/news/publications/health-matters/how-childhood-trauma-may-impact-adults

40 TNT Sports Boxing. (23 November 2020). Full fight replay: Mike Tyson v Frank Bruno. https://www.youtube.com/watch?v=jfpUia2gJjg

41 Magee, Will. (20 October 2016). The Battle Of Britain: Remembering Lennox Lewis' Epic Clash With Frank Bruno. https://www.vice.com/en/article/pgnk48/the-battle-of-britain-remembering-lennox-lewis-epic-clash-with-frank-bruno

42 Brainy Quote. Frank Bruno Quotes. https://www.brainyquote.com/quotes/frank_bruno_486279

43 Kelso, Paul. (4 November 2023). My illness could help others, says Bruno. *The Guardian*. https://www.theguardian.com/society/2003/nov/04/mentalhealth.medicineandhealth

44 Gibson, Owen. (23 September 2003). Sun on the ropes over 'Bonkers Bruno' story. *The Guardian*. https://www.theguardian.com/media/2003/sep/23/pressandpublishing.mentalhealth

45 Dawson, Alan. (9 June 2017). Yes, you can make it as a professional fighter – but only 19 athletes out of 21,000 successfully manage it. Business

Insider. https://www.businessinsider.com/mcgregor-mayweather-fight-economics-ufc-mma-bellator-boxing-paul-daley-2017-6

46 Hayes, Andy. (1 September 2022). Serena Williams announces plan to retire: 'I'm evolving away from tennis'. Sky News. https://news.sky.com/story/serena-williams-announces-plan-to-retire-im-evolving-away-from-tennis-12669136

47 Mind. Mental health crisis care services 'under-resourced, understaffed and overstretched'. https://www.mind.org.uk/news-campaigns/news/mental-health-crisis-care-services-under-resourced-understaffed-and-overstretched

48 Young, Alex. (14 July 2023). Dele Alli: Full transcript of Gary Neville interview on sexual abuse, addiction and mental health struggles. *The Standard*. https://www.standard.co.uk/sport/football/dele-alli-interview-in-full-gary-neville-b1094117.html

49 Adams, Joe. (19 July 2023). Mauricio Pochettino admits he "couldn't finish" Dele Alli's "painful" interview. https://www.sportbible.com/football/premier-league/mauricio-pochettino-dele-alli-interview-721830-20230719

50 Nightingale, Sarah. (1 August 2023). Interview with Martin Nash.

51 Ibid.

52 Dawson, Alan. (1 August 2021). Simone Biles 'really needs to check herself,' according to a former Olympic gold medalist. Business Insider. https://www.businessinsider.com/simone-biles-really-needs-to-check-herself-henry-cejudo-says-2021-8?r=US&IR=T

53 Sealey, Louis. (28 July 2021). Piers Morgan claims Simone Biles 'let her country down' after pulling out of Tokyo 2020 Olympics. *Metro*. https://metro.co.uk/2021/07/28/olympics-piers-morgan-slams-selfish-simone-biles-letting-country-down-tokyo-15000340/

54 American College of Sports Medicine. (9 August 2021). The American College of Sports Medicine Statement on Mental Health Challenges for Athletes. https://www.acsm.org/news-detail/2021/08/09/the-american-college-of-sports-medicine-statement-on-mental-health-challenges-for-athletes

55 Christian, Alex. (13 March 2023). Is it impossible to end burnout? BBC. https://www.bbc.com/worklife/article/20230309-is-it-impossible-to-end-burnout#:~:text=In%20the%20new%20world%20of,highest%20figure%20since%20May%202021

56 Sáez, Iker, Solabarrieta, Josu, and Rubio, Isabel. (26 May 2021). Reasons for Sports-Based Physical Activity Dropouts in University Students. https://www.ncbi.nlm.nih.gov/pmc/articles/PMC8198925/

57 Popoli, Maurizio, et al. (November 2011). The stressed synapse: The impact of stress and glucocorticoids on glutamate transmission. *Nature Reviews Neuroscience*. https://www.researchgate.net/publication/51840098_The_stressed_synapse_The_impact_of_stress_and_glucocorticoids_on_glutamate_transmission_Nature_reviews

58 *The Edge of Everything*. (2023). Directed by Sam Blair. Studio 99.

59 Ibid.

60 Herring, Stanley, et al. (2017). Psychological Issues Related to Illness and Injury in Athletes and the Team Physician: a Consensus Statement—2016 Update. *Current Sports Medicine Reports*, 16(3), p189–201, 5/6. https://journals.lww.com/acsm-csmr/fulltext/2017/05000/psychological_issues_related_to_illness_and_injury.18.aspx

61 Rice, Simon M., et al. (20 February 2016). The Mental Health of Elite Athletes: A Narrative Systematic Review. *Sports Med.* https://www.ncbi.nlm.nih.gov/pmc/articles/PMC4996886/

62 Grange, Dr Pippa. (2020). *Fear Less*, p6. Random House.

63 Mann, Simon. (22 August 1999). England hit an all-time low. BBC. http://news.bbc.co.uk/1/hi/sport/cricket/england_v_new_zealand/427262.stm

64 Burnton, Simon, and Martin, Ali. (19 July 2022). 'We are not cars you can fill up': Ben Stokes complains of burden on players. *The Guardian*. https://www.theguardian.com/sport/2022/jul/19/we-are-not-cars-you-can-fill-up-ben-stokes-complaints-of-burden-on-players

65 Niles, Bertram. (8 July 2020). Relief all round as cash-starved cricket returns after lockdown. https://news.cgtn.com/news/2020-07-08/Relief-all-round-as-cash-starved-cricket-returns-after-lockdown-RXEGhcT6De/index.html

66 Grange, Dr Pippa. (2020). *Fear Less*, p56. Random House.

67 In the Stiffs. (19 April 2020). Joe Hart On Fabio Capello. https://www.youtube.com/watch?v=Uf68AMuk_Yo

68 Wollaston, Sam. (17 June 2018). Managing England: The Impossible Job review – tracing 52 years of hurt. *The Guardian*. https://www.theguardian.com/tv-and-radio/2018/jun/17/managing-england-the-impossible-job-review-52-years-of-hurt

69 Barbour, Shannon. (20 January 2023). How Naomi Osaka Deals With Anxious Thoughts. https://www.wondermind.com/article/naomi-osaka-meditation/

70 Bull, Andy. (18 September 2013). 'It took 10 years to recover': the story of Scott Boswell and the yips. *The Guardian*. https://www.theguardian.com/sport/2013/sep/18/scott-boswell-and-the-yips

71 Syed, Matthew. (April 2011). *Bounce: The of Myth of Talent and the Power of Practice*, p177. Fourth Estate.

72 Syed, Matthew. (April 2011). *Bounce: The of Myth of Talent and the Power of Practice*, p186. Fourth Estate.

73 O'Neal, Lonnae. (12 April 2017). Derrick Rose hates fame, but still hopes to be an NBA champion. https://andscape.com/features/derrick-rose-nba-new-york-knicks-free-agency

74 Csikszentmihalyi, Mihaly. (1990). *Flow*, p73. Rider.

75 Harrell, Eben. (30 October 2015). How 1% Performance Improvements Led to Olympic Gold. *Harvard Business Review*. https://hbr.org/2015/10/how-1-performance-improvements-led-to-olympic-gold

76 Jones, Jason, et al. (1 February 2019). Association between late-night tweeting and next-day game performance among professional basketball

players. *Science Direct – Sleep health*. https://www.sciencedirect.com/science/article/abs/pii/S2352721818301724

77 The Associated Press. (23 October 2012). Number of active users at Facebook over the years. https://www.yahoo.com/news/number-active-users-facebook-over-230449748.html

78 Reed, Jesse. (24 July 2012). Olympic Swimming 2012: Twitter Misadventures of Australian Star Stephanie Rice. Bleacher Report. https://bleacherreport.com/articles/1269573-olympic-swimming-2012-twitter-misadventures-of-australian-star-stephanie-rice

79 Ottesen, Didrik. (30 July 2012). London 2012 Olympics: Australian swimmer Emily Seebohm blames Twitter and Facebook for failure. *The Telegraph*. https://www.telegraph.co.uk/sport/olympics/news/9440774/London-2012-Olympics-Australian-swimmer-Emily-Seebohm-blames-Twitter-and-Facebook-for-failure.html

80 Ford, JL, et al. (27 October 2017). Sport-related anxiety: current insights. *Open Access Journal of Sports Medicine*. https://www.dovepress.com/sport-related-anxiety-current-insights-peer-reviewed-fulltext-article-OAJSM

81 Andrews, Luke. (26 April 2023). Running 5 miles as punishment for eating a cookie: How social media is fueling eating disorders among female athletes, according to research. *Daily Mail*. https://www.dailymail.co.uk/health/article-12013099/Running-5-miles-eating-cookie-Social-media-eating-disorders-female-athletes.html

82 Shirole, Thrupti. (4 May 2023). Spring Forward: Breaking Free from Unrealistic Body Standards in Women's Sports. MedIndia. https://www.medindia.net/news/healthwatch/spring-forward-empowering-female-athletes-with-healthy-habits-and-positive-body-image-211631-1.htm

83 Malik, Aisha. (18 April 2023). YouTube updates its policies on eating disorder content, will ban videos showing 'imitable behavior'. https://techcrunch.com/2023/04/18/youtube-updates-its-policies-on-eating-disorder-content-will-ban-videos-showing-imitable-behavior/

84 CBC Sports. (11 September 2019). Female Aussie footballer, trolled for photo of her in mid-kick, gets statue in response." https://www.cbc.ca/sports/tayla-harris-afl-statue-australia-1.5279580

85 Women's Agenda. (19 March 2019). The trolls came so the photo of Tayla Harris was removed. Now it's being widely celebrated. https://womensagenda.com.au/latest/the-trolls-came-so-7afl-removed-the-photo-of-tayla-harris-now-its-being-widely-celebrated/

86 John, Anna, et al. (19 April 2018). Self-Harm, Suicidal Behaviours, and Young People: Systematic Review. *Journal of Medical Internet Research*. https://www.jmir.org/2018/4/e129/

87 Sweney, Mark. (1 August 2022). England's Euros triumph draws record TV audience of 17m. *The Guardian*. https://www.theguardian.com/football/2022/aug/01/england-victory-in-womens-euro-2022-final-draws-record-tv-audience-of-17m

88 Statista Research Department. (9 December 2022). Share of women's soccer fans worldwide in 2019, by gender. https://www.statista.com/statistics/1134070/women-soccer-fans-gender/
89 Grange, Dr Pippa. (2020). *Fear Less*, p226. Random House.
90 Pesce, Nicole Lyn. (13 July 2019). The U.S. women's team won the World Cup, and they're about to get paid — by sponsors, anyway. https://www.marketwatch.com/story/us-womens-soccer-won-the-world-cup-and-theyre-about-to-get-paid-by-sponsors-anyway-2019-07-09
91 Tennery, Amy. (24 March 2021) 'We have filled stadiums': U.S. soccer star Rapinoe renews call for gender pay equity. Reuters. https://www.reuters.com/article/us-employment-equalpay-idUSKBN2BG2F1
92 Jacobs, Shahida. (18 August 2020). WTA stars dominate 2020 Forbes Highest-Paid Female Athletes list as Naomi Osaka leads Serena Williams. https://www.tennis365.com/wta-tour/wta-stars-dominate-2020-forbes-highest-paid-female-athletes-list-as-naomi-osaka-leads-serena-williams/
93 Mench, Chris. (16 May 2023). Serena Williams Is the Only Woman Ranking Among the World's Highest-Paid Athletes This Year. *Men's Journal.* https://www.mensjournal.com/news/serena-williams-highest-paid-female-athlete-2023
94 Daniel, Richard, and Cooper, Pete. (2 August 2022). Women's football: 'I'm a pro footballer but I have a second job'. BBC. https://www.bbc.co.uk/news/uk-england-suffolk-62386612
95 Beals, K A, and Manore, M M. (June 1994). The prevalence and consequences of subclinical eating disorders in female athletes. *International Journal of Sport Nutrition and Exercise Metabolism.* https://pubmed.ncbi.nlm.nih.gov/8054962/
96 Holmes, Lindsay. (26 April 2019). Serena Williams Gets Real About Managing Anxiety. HuffPost. https://www.huffingtonpost.co.uk/entry/serena-williams-anxiety-motherhood_n_5ae1d4fbe4b02baed1b76a51
97 Women in Football. https://www.womeninfootball.co.uk/
98 Grange, Dr Pippa. (2020). *Fear Less*, p67. Random House.
99 Reuters. (30 December 2020). 'Promoted because of COVID'? Leeds hit back at pundit. https://www.reuters.com/article/sports/promoted-because-of-covid-leeds-hit-back-at-pundit-idUSKBN2940PF/
100 Cheshire, Tom. (15 July 2023). Why are women footballers facing an 'epidemic' of ACL injuries? Sky News. https://news.sky.com/story/an-epidemic-of-acl-injuries-affecting-women-footballers-but-why-is-it-happening-12921045
101 Wolanin, Andrew, et al. (2015). Depression in Athletes Prevalence and Risk Factors. *Current Sports Medicine Reports.* https://vincerainstitute.com/why-vincera/news-articles/files/015-Depression_in_Athletes___Prevalence_and_Risk.pdf
102 Gulliver, A, et al. (29 April 2014). The mental health of Australian elite athletes. *Journal of Science and Medicine in Sport.* https://pubmed.ncbi.nlm.nih.gov/24882147/

103 Foster, Richard. (16 January 2017). What do footballers do while recovering from long-term injuries? *The Guardian*. https://www.theguardian.com/football/the-agony-and-the-ecstasy/2017/jan/16/footballers-long-term-injuries-gundogan-manchester-city

104 Joynson, Danielle. (20 January 2015). Mark Cavendish angrily responds to journalist by asking if wife is cheating on him. https://www.sportsmole.co.uk/off-the-pitch/news/cavendish-asks-journalist-if-wife-is-cheating_200118.html

105 *Mark Cavendish: Never Enough*. (2023). Directed by Alex Kiehl.

106 Ostanek, Dani. (3 July 2024). 'Disbelief', gratitude, and family – Mark Cavendish celebrates a record-breaking Tour de France sprint win. https://www.cyclingnews.com/news/mark-cavendish-cements-legendary-status-as-cyclings-most-successful-sprinter/

107 Didehbani, Nyaz, et al. (August 2013). Depressive Symptoms and Concussions in Aging Retired NFL Players. *Archives of Clinical Neuropsychology*. https://www.ncbi.nlm.nih.gov/pmc/articles/PMC4007104/

108 Alzheimer's Association. Chronic Traumatic Encephalopathy (CTE). https://www.alz.org/alzheimers-dementia/what-is-dementia/related_conditions/chronic-traumatic-encephalopathy

109 Most, Doug. (7 February 2023). BU Finds CTE in Nearly 92 Percent of Ex-NFL Players Studied. https://www.bu.edu/articles/2023/bu-finds-cte-in-nearly-92-percent-of-former-nfl-players-studied/

110 Boston University Chobanian & Avedisian School of Medicine. (6 February 2023). Researchers Find CTE in 345 of 376 Former NFL Players Studied. https://www.bumc.bu.edu/busm/2023/02/06/researchers-find-cte-in-345-of-376-former-nfl-players-studied

111 Boston University CTE Center. (21 September 2017). BU CTE Center Statement on Aaron Hernandez. https://www.bu.edu/cte/2017/09/21/bu-cte-center-statement-on-aaron-hernandez/

112 Gonzales, Richard. (9 November 2017). Researcher Says Aaron Hernandez's Brain Showed Signs Of Severe CTE. NPR. https://www.npr.org/sections/thetwo-way/2017/11/09/563194252/researcher-says-aaron-hernandez-s-brain-showed-signs-of-severe-cte

113 Associated Press. (9 November 2017). New images show Aaron Hernandez suffered from extreme case of CTE. https://www.theguardian.com/sport/2017/nov/09/aaron-hernandez-cte-brain-damage-photos

114 Bull, Andy. (8 December 2020). Steve Thompson: 'I can't remember winning the World Cup'. *The Guardian*. https://www.theguardian.com/sport/2020/dec/08/steve-thompson-interview-world-cup-rugby-union-dementia-special-report

115 Shaffer, Leah. (13 January 2020). Should Parents Be Afraid To Let Their Kids Play Football? Five Thirty Eight. https://fivethirtyeight.com/features/should-parents-be-afraid-to-let-their-kids-play-football/#:~:text=Though%20parents%20are%20responding%20to,of%20existence%2C%20at%20any%20level

116 Jacobs, Shaun. (6 May 2023). Most valuable sports franchises in the world. *Daily Investor*. https://dailyinvestor.com/world/15470/most-valuable-sports-franchises-in-the-world/
117 Abdalazem, Reem. (28 April 2023). Who is the lowest paid player in the NFL? Is there a minimum salary in American football? https://en.as.com/nfl/who-is-the-lowest-paid-player-in-the-nfl-is-there-a-minimum-salary-in-american-football-n-2
118 ESPN. (5 August 2024). Highest-paid NFL players: Most guaranteed money at every position. https://www.espn.co.uk/nfl/story/_/id/34096853/highest-paid-nfl-players-tracking-most-money-guaranteed-per-year-every-position
119 *The Guardian*. (14 November 2009). Robert Enke's father reveals history of his son's depression. https://www.theguardian.com/football/2009/nov/14/robert-enke-father-depression-germany
120 BBC News. (9 November 2021). Man City did not give 'right support' to teenager, inquest told. https://www.bbc.co.uk/news/uk-england-manchester-59214647
121 Cunningham, Sam. (7 January 2022). Premier League reveal 97% of players who come through top academies never play a minute of top-flight football. https://inews.co.uk/sport/football/premier-league-academy-players-figures-appearances-numbers-1387302
122 Barlow, Eleanor, and Johnson, Helen. (17 November 2020). Inquest opens into tragic death of former Manchester City youth player Jeremy Wisten. *Manchester Evening News*. https://www.manchestereveningnews.co.uk/news/greater-manchester-news/inquest-opens-tragic-death-former-19293474
123 Nightingale, Sarah. (1 August 2023). Interview with Martin Nash.
124 Ibid.
125 Wills, Juliette. (26 August 2020). Why football no longer agrees with Bill Shankly. *The Guardian*. https://www.theguardian.com/football/2002/aug/26/sport.comment1
126 Steinberg, Jacob. (7 March 2014). The Joy of Six: football quotes. *The Guardian*. https://www.theguardian.com/sport/blog/2014/mar/07/joy-of-six-football-quotes
127 Pender, Matt. (10 March 2023). *Steroid Use in the WWE: Candid Truth by Hulk Hogan, The Rock and More*. https://prowrestlingstories.com/pro-wrestling-stories/steroid-use-wwe/
128 *Dark Side of the Ring*. Season 2, Episode 1 – Chris Benoit, Part One. Vice TV.
129 O'Connor, Anahad. (18 July 2007). Wrestler Found to Have Taken Testosterone. *The New York Times*. https://www.nytimes.com/2007/07/18/us/18wrestler.html
130 *Dark Side of the Ring*. Season 2, Episode 2 – Chris Benoit Part Two. Vice TV.
131 Ibid.

132 BBC Sport. State of Sport 2018: Half of retired sportspeople have concerns over mental and emotional wellbeing. https://www.bbc.co.uk/sport/42871491
133 Ibid.
134 Sicoli, Michael. (23 February 2021). Remember Vincent Jackson. *The Quinnipiac Chronicle*. https://quchronicle.com/72204/opinion/remember-vincent-jackson/
135 Syed, Matthew. (April 2011). *Bounce: The of Myth of Talent and the Power of Practice*, p140. Fourth Estate.
136 Abu, Howa O, et al. (4 October 2019). Religious practices and long-term survival after hospital discharge for an acute coronary syndrome. *PLOS One*. https://www.ncbi.nlm.nih.gov/pmc/articles/PMC6777785/
137 Syed, Matthew. (April 2011). *Bounce: The of Myth of Talent and the Power of Practice*, p142. Fourth Estate.
138 Grey-Thompson, Tanni. (April 2017). Duty of Care in Sport. https://www.gov.uk/government/publications/duty-of-care-in-sport-review
139 Society for Sport, Exercise & Performance Psychology. (May 2016). Career Transitions in Sport. https://www.apadivisions.org/division-47/publications/sportpsych-works/career-transitions.pdf
140 Kandola, Aaron. (18 January 2024). How to increase serotonin with or without medication. https://www.medicalnewstoday.com/articles/how-to-increase-serotonin
141 Cole, Bill. (1998). Stress Of Transitions In Life And Sport. https://www.mentalgamecoach.com/the-stress-of-transitions-in-life-and-sport-how-both-stressors-impact-your-performance
142 Buckmaster, Luke. (28 February 2017). Ian Thorpe on bullying, depression and athletes' mental health. *The Guardian*. https://www.theguardian.com/tv-and-radio/2017/mar/01/ian-thorpe-on-bullying-depression-and-athletes-mental-health
143 McRae, Donald. (12 November 2012). Ian Thorpe: "I was surrounded by people but had this intense loneliness". *The Guardian*. https://www.theguardian.com/sport/2012/nov/12/ian-thorpe-swimming-depression
144 Walters, Matt. (20 January 2022). Ian Thorpe Reveals the Lessons he has Learned Living With Depression. https://www.adidas-group.com/en/magazine/behind-the-scenes/ian-thorpe-reveals-the-lessons-he-has-learned-living-with-depression
145 Wikipedia. List of athletes who competed in both the Summer and Winter Olympic games. https://en.wikipedia.org/wiki/List_of_athletes_who_competed_in_both_the_Summer_and_Winter_Olympic_games
146 Williams, Serena. (9 August 2022). Serena Williams Says Farewell to Tennis On Her Own Terms–And In Her Own Words. *Vogue*. https://www.vogue.com/article/serena-williams-retirement-in-her-own-words
147 MacInnes, Paul. (16 May 2022). Jake Daniels becomes first UK male footballer to come out as gay since 1990. *The Guardian*. https://www.

theguardian.com/football/2022/may/16/jake-daniels-becomes-first-uk-male-footballer-to-come-out-as-gay-since-1990

148 Statista Research Department. (9 December 2022). Countries with the most professional soccer players worldwide as of 2023. https://www.statista.com/statistics/1283927/number-pro-soccer-players-by-country/

149 Rey, Ezequiel, et al. (June 2022). No sport for old players. A longitudinal study of aging effects on match performance in elite soccer. *Journal of Science and Medicine in Sport.* https://www.sciencedirect.com/science/article/pii/S1440244022000469

150 Office for National Statistics. (27 May 2021). Sexual orientation, UK: 2019. https://www.ons.gov.uk/peoplepopulationandcommunity/culturalidentity/sexuality/bulletins/sexualidentityuk/2019

151 Clough, Brian. (1995). *Clough: The Autobiography*, p319. Corgi Adult.

152 Grange, Dr Pippa. (2020). *Fear Less*, p54. Random House.

153 Stroude, Will. (22 October 2020). How homophobia claimed the life and career of Justin Fashanu, the world's first openly gay footballer. *Attitude.* https://www.attitude.co.uk/culture/sexuality/how-homophobia-claimed-the-life-and-career-of-justin-fashanu-the-worlds-first-openly-gay-footballer-301868/

154 Nightingale, Sarah. (1 August 2023). Interview with Martin Nash.

155 Syed, Matthew. (April 2011). *Bounce: The of Myth of Talent and the Power of Practice,* p186. Fourth Estate.

156 Bethune, Sophie. (January 2019). Gen Z more likely to report mental health concerns. *Monitor on Psychology.* https://www.apa.org/monitor/2019/01/gen-z

157 Davis, Maggie. (21 February 2023). Gen Zers Nearly 3 Times More Likely Than Older Generations To Seek Therapy Since Start of Pandemic. https://www.valuepenguin.com/therapy-survey

158 Office of National Statistics. (19 December 2023). Suicides in England and Wales: 2022 registrations. https://www.ons.gov.uk/peoplepopulationandcommunity/birthsdeathsandmarriages/deaths/bulletins/suicidesintheunitedkingdom/2022registrations

159 Parker, Kim, and Igielnik, Ruth. (14 May 2020). On the Cusp of Adulthood and Facing an Uncertain Future: What We Know About Gen Z So Far. Pew Research. https://www.pewresearch.org/social-trends/2020/05/14/on-the-cusp-of-adulthood-and-facing-an-uncertain-future-what-we-know-about-gen-z-so-far-2/

160 GLAAD. (30 March 2017). Accelerating Acceptance: GLAAD Study Reveals Twenty Percent of Millennials Identify as LGBTQ. https://glaad.org/releases/new-glaad-study-reveals-twenty-percent-millennials-identify-lgbtq/

161 Milton, Josh. (15 August 2022). UK Anti-LGBTQ+ hate crime reports explode across UK, damning police figures confirm. https://www.thepinknews.com/2022/08/15/anti-lgbtq-hate-crime-police-uk/

162 Bartucca, Julie. (16 March 2018). The Most Complicated Object in the Universe. UConn Communications. https://today.uconn.edu/2018/03/complicated-object-universe/

163 Higgs, John. (2015). *Stranger Than We Can Imagine – Making Sense of the Twentieth Century*, p18. Hachette UK.

164 Kurzweil, Ray, et all. (1999). *The Age of Spiritual Machines*. Viking.

TRIGGERHUB IS ONE OF THE MOST ELITE AND SCIENTIFICALLY PROVEN FORMS OF MENTAL HEALTH INTERVENTION

Trigger Publishing is the leading independent mental health and wellbeing publisher in the UK and US. Our collection of bibliotherapeutic books and the power of lived experience change lives forever. Our courageous authors' lived experiences and the power of their stories are scientifically endorsed by independent federal, state and privately funded research in the US. These stories are intrinsic elements in reducing stigma, making those with poor mental health feel less alone, giving them the privacy they need to heal, ensuring they are guided by the essential steps to kick-start their own journeys to recovery, and providing hope and inspiration when they need it most.

Clinical and scientific research conducted by assistant professor Dr Kristin Kosyluk and her highly acclaimed team in the Department of Mental Health Law & Policy at the University of South Florida (USF), as well as complementary research by her peers across the US, has independently verified the power of lived experience as a core component in achieving mental health prosperity. Their findings categorically confirm lived experience as a leading method in treating those struggling with poor mental health by significantly reducing stigma and the time it takes for them to seek help, self-help or signposting if they are struggling.

Delivered through TriggerHub, our unique online portal and smartphone app, we make our library of bibliotherapeutic titles and other vital resources accessible to individuals and organizations anywhere, at any time and with complete privacy, a crucial element of recovery. As such, TriggerHub is the primary recommendation across the UK and US for the delivery of lived experiences.

At Trigger Publishing and TriggerHub, we proudly lead the way in making the unseen become seen. We are dedicated to humanizing mental health, breaking stigma and challenging outdated societal values to create real action and impact. Find out more about our world-leading work with lived experience and bibliotherapy via triggerhub.com, or by joining us on:

- @triggerhub_
- @triggerhub.org
- @triggerhub_

Dr Kristin Kosyluk, PhD, is an assistant professor in the Department of Mental Health Law & Policy at USF, a faculty affiliate of the Louis de la Parte Florida Mental Health Institute, and director of the STigma Action Research (STAR) Lab. Find out more about Dr Kristin Kosyluk, her team and their work by visiting:

USF Department of Mental Health Law & Policy:
www.usf.edu/cbcs/mhlp/index.aspx

USF College of Behavioral and Community Sciences:
www.usf.edu/cbcs/index.aspx

STAR Lab: www.usf.edu/cbcs/mhlp/centers/star-lab/

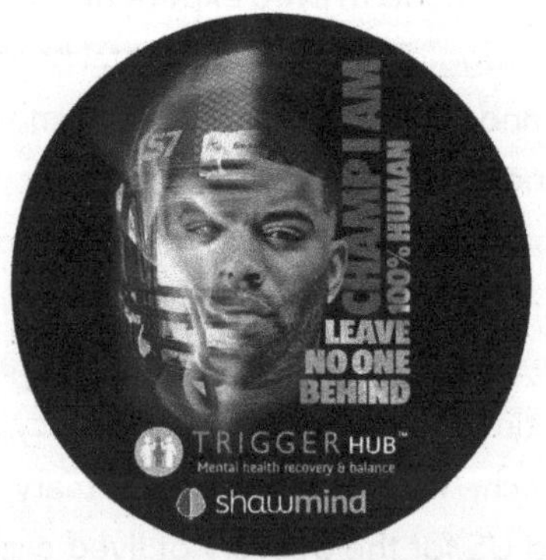

For more information, visit BJ-Super7.com